T0127756

Clinical Diagnosis in

PHYSICAL MEDICINE
& REHABILITATION

CASE BY CASE

Clinical Diagnosis in
PHYSICAL MEDICINE
& REHABILITATION

CASE BY CASE

Subhadra Nori, MD
Regional Medical Director
Department of Rehabilitation Medicine;
Attending Physiatrist
Elmhurst and Queens Hospital Centers;
Clinical Associate Professor
Icahn School of Medicine, Mount Sinai
New York, NY

Michelle Stern, MD
Chairman of the Department of Rehabilitation Medicine
Health & Hospital Jacobi and North Central Bronx;
Clinical Associate Professor
Albert Einstein College of Medicine
New York, NY

Se Won Lee, MD
Residency Program Director
Department of Physical Medicine and Rehabilitation
Mountain View Medical Center
Las Vegas, NV

ELSEVIER

Elsevier
1600 John F. Kennedy Blvd.
Ste 1800
Philadelphia, PA 19103-2899

CLINICAL DIAGNOSIS IN PHYSICAL MEDICINE & REHABILITATION,
FIRST EDITION

ISBN: 978-0-323-72084-7

Copyright © 2022 by Elsevier, Inc. All rights reserved.

No part of this publication may be reproduced or transmitted in any form or by any means, electronic or mechanical, including photocopying, recording, or any information storage and retrieval system, without permission in writing from the publisher. Details on how to seek permission, further information about the Publisher's permissions policies and our arrangements with organizations such as the Copyright Clearance Center and the Copyright Licensing Agency, can be found at our website: www.elsevier.com/permissions.

This book and the individual contributions contained in it are protected under copyright by the Publisher (other than as may be noted herein)

Notice

Practitioners and researchers must always rely on their own experience and knowledge in evaluating and using any information, methods, compounds or experiments described herein. Because of rapid advances in the medical sciences, in particular, independent verification of diagnoses and drug dosages should be made. To the fullest extent of the law, no responsibility is assumed by Elsevier, authors, editors or contributors for any injury and/or damage to persons or property as a matter of products liability, negligence or otherwise, or from any use or operation of any methods, products, instructions, or ideas contained in the material herein.

ISBN: 978-0-323-72084-7

Content Strategist: Humayra R. Khan
Content Development Manager: Ellen Wurm-Cutter
Content Development Specialist: Dominque McPherson
Publishing Services Manager: Shereen Jameel
Project Manager: Nadhiya Sekar
Design Direction: Renee Duenow

Printed in the United States

Last digit is the print number: 9 8 7 6 5 4 3 2 1

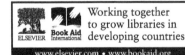

Working together
to grow libraries in
developing countries

www.elsevier.com • www.bookaid.org

Dr. Eric Aguila, MD
Physiatrist
Department of Rehabilitation
VA Southern Nevada Healthcare System
Las Vegas, Nevada

Dr. Mohammed Emam, MD
Assistant Professor
Department of Orthopaedics and
    Rehabilitation Medicine
Associate Program Director
Division of Sports Medicine
SUNY Downstate Medical Center
Brooklyn, New York

Dr. Jasmine H. Harris, MD
Resident Physician
Department of Rehabilitation Medicine and
    Human Performance
Icahn School of Medicine, Mount Sinai
New York, New York

Dr. Maryam Hosseini, MD
PM&R Resident Physician
Department of Physical Medicine and
    Rehabilitation
Montefiore Medical Center
Albert Einstein College of Medicine
The Bronx, New York

Dr. Se Won Lee, MD
Residency Program Director
Department of Physical Medicine and
    Rehabilitation
Mountain View Medical Center
Las Vegas, NV

Dr. Patrick Mahaney, MD, MS, FAAPMR
Associate Medical Director
Mountain Valley Regional Rehabilitation
    Hospital
Prescott Valley, Arizona

Dr. Vivek Nagar, MD, M.B.A.
Department of Rehabilitation Medicine
Montefiore Medical Center
Albert Einstein School of Medicine
The Bronx, New York

Dr. Reina Nakamura, DO
Assistant Professor
Department of Physical Medicine and
    Rehabilitation
University of Michigan
Ann Arbor, Michigan

Dr. Subhadra Nori, MD
Regional Medical Director
Department of Rehabilitation Medicine
Attending Physiatrist
Elmhurst and Queens Hospital Centers
Clinical Associate Professor
Icahn School of Medicine, Mount Sinai
New York, NY

Dr. Kishan A. Sitapara, MD
Resident Physician
Department of Physical Medicine and
    Rehabilitation
Montefiore Medical Center
Albert Einstein School of Medicine
The Bronx, New York

Dr. Michelle Stern, MD
Chairman of the Department of
    Rehabilitation Medicine
Health & Hospital Jacobi and North Central
    Bronx
Clinical Associate Professor
Albert Einstein College of Medicine
New York, NY

Dr. Iris Tian, DO
Resident Physician
Department of Rehabilitation Medicine and
    Human Performance
Icahn School of Medicine, Mount Sinai
New York, New York

Dr. Lynn D. Weiss, MD
Chairman
Department of Physical Medicine and
    Rehabilitation
NYU Winthrop Hospital
Mineola, New York

Physical medicine and rehabilitation has many sectors. Musculoskeletal medicine is only one part. The practice of musculoskeletal medicine involves both art and science. It is a skill that physicians develop over time. A solid foundation laid from the beginning of the medical courses is essential to master this skill. The intention of this book is to provide an overview of the most frequently seen conditions in everyday physiatry practice.

An attempt was made to provide comprehensive information but science is constantly evolving and information changes rapidly. This book is intended to provide guidance to all levels of learning from student to an independent practitioner.

CONTENTS

ACKNOWLEDGEMENTS

First, I want to thank my husband, Dr. D. Nori, who has been my life partner for 40+ years and has guided me at every step of my career and life. Second, I would like to thank Teresita Pascua who made my transcripts readable. Third, I would like to thank all the contributing authors. Fourth, I owe the production of this book to the editorial staff at Elsevier, Ms. Dominque McPherson. Fifth, I want to thank all my patients from whom I learned a lot. Finally, I would like to thank Dr. Shuvendu Sen whose book *Principles of Clinical Diagnosis Case by Case* was the inspiration for this project.

Subhadra Nori

I want to thank my wife, Hyunjoo, and my daughter, Jane, for their patience while preparing for this book. I would like to thank my mentors, Dr. Dennis DJ Kim and Dr. Mooyeon Oh-Park, for their teaching. I thank my residents and colleagues who inspire me constantly. Lastly, I want to thank Dr. Nori and everyone who made this publication possible.

Se Won Lee

CHAPTER 1

Neck Pain

Dr. Subhadra Nori, MD

Case History

A 57-year-old woman presents to the Physical Medicine and Rehabilitation (PM&R) clinic with a history of neck pain. She describes her pain as constant. She experiences pain on movement of the neck. This pain has been present for about 4 to 5 months and is progressively worsening. She takes an occasional Tylenol which seems to help but temporarily. There is numbness of the upper left arm; she is unable to sleep because of this pain. She has not seen any other physician nor had any workup.

 Past medical history: She has history of hypertension (HTN) for which she is on Losartan, 25 mg. O.D. for the past 10 years. She is postmenopausal.

 Social history: She works as a school teacher, lives with family in an apartment with elevator on the fourth floor. She has two children aged 18 and 16 years.

 Past surgical history: None

 Allergies: Dust

 Medications: Losartan, 25 mg O.D., occasional Tylenol

 BP: 140/70 mmHg, RR: 14/min, PR: 75 pm, Temp: 97° F, Ht: 5'5, Wt: 130 lbs, BMI: 22 kg/m²

PHYSICAL EXAMINATION

 Well-developed (WD), well-nourished (WN) lady in moderate distress.

 Head, ears, eyes, nose and throat (HEENT): Extraocular movement (EOM)'s full, no ptosis.

 General: She is alert, oriented and in mild to moderate distress because of L sided neck pain.

 Extremities: No edema, no skin rashes, no surgical scars, no fasciculations seen

 Musculoskeletal examination: Range of motion (ROM) of neck—complete in all directions.

MOTOR EXAMINATION

 Right upper extremity (RUE) all groups 5/5 left upper extremity (LUE) 3/5 deltoid, biceps, and brachioradialis.

 All other muscles were 5/5.

 There was some wasting of deltoid and biceps muscles.

 Deep tendon reflex (DTR)-1+ in biceps, brachioradialis on L 2 and + on R

 Sensory examination: Dull to light touch in lateral forearm on the LUE intact in all dermatomes on the RUE.

 Gait was within normal limits (WNL) without any deviations.

 Tone was normal.

 Labs: White blood cell (WBC) 7000, cell/mL; hemoglobin 12.0 g/dL.

General Discussion

General approach to neck pain. The approach to a patient with subacute onset neck pain is uniquely different from that of acute pain. The initial focus should be to differentiate neurologic disorders from musculoskeletal conditions. The points to focus in the physical examination are muscle wasting of deltoid and biceps. Weakness of muscle supplied by the C5–C6 roots and depressed reflexes in the C5–C6 distribution. Sensory loss also conforms to this distribution.

 Differential diagnosis should include:

1. **Discogenic pain**—acute disc herniation at cervical spine intervertebral joints can lead to nerve root compression.

Symptoms depend upon the level of compression. A herniated nucleus pulposus (HNP) at C4–C5 will be compressing C5 root causing arm pain, tingling, and root burning that may radiate to fingertips. Muscles supplied (diagram C spine, nerves by root) C5 nerve, that is, deltoid. Therefore a patient with HNP at C4–C5 will have neurologic symptoms affecting C5 nerve root. Biceps, brachioradialis, and coracobrachialis will be affected (Fig. 1.1).

2. **Compression fracture**—history of trauma usually precedes. Examination reveals pain and tenderness at spine level worsening with flexion. Compression fracture can be caused by traumatic or nontraumatic causes.

3. **Strains and strains**—diffuse neck pain following a motor accident vehicle usually referred to as "whiplash." Examination is positive for neck tenderness diffusely, usually no neurologic symptoms exist.

4. **Osteoarthritis/spondylosis**—refer to generalized osteoarthritis (OA) in an elderly patient, usually pain is worse with activity. Flexion may cause more pain than extension. Neurologic symptoms are seen in the distribution of nerve root that is compromised.

5. **Connective tissue disease**—multiple joint arthralgia, fever, weight loss, fatigue and other systemic symptoms are seen. Examination reveals spinous process tenderness and other joint tenderness.

6. **Inflammatory spondylarthropathies**—present as neck pain with intermittent pain, morning stiffness worsening with activity.

7. **Malignancy**—constant pain, worsen in supine position. Systemic manifestation, such as weight loss, may accompany.

8. **Vertebral discitis**—constant pain, often no fever, normal blood count but C-reactive protein (CRP) and erythrocyte sedimentation rate (ESR) are frequently elevated.

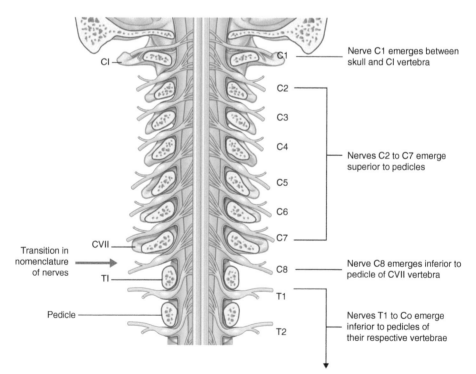

Fig. 1.1 Nomenclature of spinal nerves, posterior view. (From R.L. Drake, W. Vogl, A.W.M. Mitchell. Gray's Anatomy for Students, 4e. Elsevier, Philadelphia, 2020, Fig. 1.25.)

9. **Cervical myelopathy**—present in 90% of individuals by the seventh decade and is the most common form of spinal cord dysfunction in people over 55 years of age. Upper motor neuron signs and symptoms.

    Referred pain: lung cancer—both small cell and adenocarcinoma can metastasize to cervical spine and cause epidural or extradural metastasis, likewise breast cancer can metastasize to cervical spine.

10. **Cervical myeloradiculopathy**—believed to occur because of spondylosis and repetitive compression damage to C-spinal cord and roots.[1] Anterior spondylitic spurs, posterior longitudinal ligament in folding can also cause compression. Acute flexion extension injuries can initiate compression of an already compromised C-spine because of spurs, osteophytes, and thickening of ligaments.

    Signs and symptoms are characterized by weakness in lower extremities, gait disturbances. Spasticity and upper motor neuron changes caused by corticospinal and spinocerebellar tract dysfunction. Additional sign and symptoms, such as pain in upper C-spine, tingling, numbness and paresthesia in fingers, and sensory changes, can also manifest. Occasional bowel and bladder changes can be seen depending on compression level.[2]

    Myeloradiculopathy: combination of myelopathy and radiculopathy, a clinically complex clinical presentation.[3] Typically, patients present with radicular symptoms, that is, pain and weakness in the arms combined with myelopathy symptoms in the legs, that is, gait disturbance, loss of position, and vibration sense and spasticity. Sometimes signs and symptoms overlap.

11. **Referred pain because of bony metastasis**—many cancers can metastasize to cervical vertebrae. The prime examples are lung cancer both small cell and adenocarcinomas, thyroid, breast, prostate. Both epidural and extradural compressions are possible and cause symptoms of cord compression.

12. **Motor neuron diseases** (MND)—term used to describe a group of sporadically acquired and familial disorders that affect the anterior horn cells. This group includes spinal muscular atrophy (SMA), amyotrophic lateral sclerosis (ALS), primary lateral sclerosis (PLS), progressive muscular atrophy (PMA), and progressive bulbar palsy (PBP). ALS is by far the most common with a prevalence rate of 5 to 7 per 100,000. It most commonly affects people between the age of 50 and 60 years. This disease can show signs and symptoms of both upper motor neuron (UMN) and lower motor neuron (LMN) involvement. Depending upon whether the presentation is primarily UMN, LMN, bulbar, or mixed UMN and LMN involvement, clinically patients may have weakness of upper extremity (UE), bulbar muscle weakness, that is, speech and swallowing deficits, and generalized weakness. Physical examination findings include weakness of UE muscles, hyperreflexia, fasciculations, and pathologic reflexes as Babinski and Hoffman. Tongue may also show fasciculations and atrophy.

13. **Neck tension syndrome**—a patient with this syndrome usually complains of aching discomfort at the base of the neck and upper back. Headaches may be reported if suboccipital and trapezius are involved. Referred pain may also be felt in upper arms, elbows, and forearms. Physical usually is negative. Skilled palpation techniques may help to identify the areas of trigger points. Postural biomechanics is the mainstay of management.

Case Discussion

Our patient describes indolent development of symptoms over a few months suggesting chronicity. Existence of pain with numbness in C5–C6 dermatomes, combined with weakness of deltoid, biceps, brachioradialis, and triceps muscles along with reduced reflexes, points to neurologic involvement. Therefore our focus should be on those conditions that lead to probable compression of the C5–C6 and possibly C7 roots, such as discogenic disease, spondylosis, spondylarthropathies, space occupying lesions, and metastatic compression fractures leading to nerve root compression.

Vertebral discitis is probably not a possibility because ESR and CRP are normal, likewise inflammatory arthropathies and connective tissue disorders are unlikely because the complaints are focal and multijoint involvement is not there.

Objective Data

Complete blood count—WNL
Coagulation panel—WNL
Complete metabolic panel—WNL
Complete chest x-ray (CXR)—negative for infiltrates, or any other lesions
X-ray of spine—degenerative disc, disease C4–C5 and C5–C6 disc spaces with lateral canal narrowing at C6–C7 levels, no fracture or dislocation was seen. No sclerotic or lytic lesion are seen
Magnetic resonance imaging (MRI) of C-spine—spinal root compression at C5, C6, C7 with no signal abnormality or evidence of cord compression
Electromyography (EMG) showed acute radiculopathy involving C5–C6 with preservation of motor units

Case Discussion

The aforementioned laboratory and imaging data are helpful to further narrow down the differential diagnosis. Because basal ESR and metabolic panel are normal, infection processes and discitis could be eliminated. Imaging did not reveal any lytic or blastic lesions, therefore metastatic disease can be ruled out. Also imaging was helpful to rule out traumatic involvement of C-spine, such as acute fractures and dislocation. Likewise, cord compression can be eliminated because no signal changes are seen on MRI. Clinically myelopathy was low on the suspicion index because the patient did not present with any UMN signs or symptoms, such as increased tone, positive Hoffman sign, ataxia, bladder bowel compromise, or hyperactive reflexes.

The objective data are notable for x-ray and MRI findings of disc degenerative disease at multiple levels. The C5 root compression leads to weakness of deltoid. C6 root compression is causing her weakness in biceps, brachioradialis, and decreased biceps and BR reflexes. EMG nerve conduction data are consistent with the clinical suspicion of cervical radiculopathy involving C5 and C6 roots.

Review of Proposed Pathology and Pathobiomechanics

Myelopathy, radiculopathy, and myeloradiculopathy involve structural abnormalities and lead to problems with movements. Disc height loss because of degenerative changes and dehydration lead to reduction of space both at the central canal where spinal cord is situated and lateral canal recesses where the nerve root exits. Structural changes at the discs ligaments and capsule lead to viscoelastic changes and movement abnormalities.[4] According to Wilson, flexion and extension movement cause a variety of neurologic abnormalities in severe degenerative conditions.[5]

Because of the enfolding ligaments during extension, spinal canal shortens and causes canal encroachment; disc may bulge posteriorly, further reducing space. Reduction in ROM of spine and symptoms of root compression and pain ensue.

Cervical myelopathy on the other hand is hallmarked by multilevel stenosis and encroachment of spinal cord leading to upper motor neuron findings. This encroachment is from sagittal narrowing of the canal, often by (1) osteophytes, secondary to degeneration of intervertebral joints, (2) stiffening of connective tissue, such as ligamentum flavum, (3) degeneration of intervertebral disc with bony changes, or (4) other degenerative connective tissue changes.[6]

Structural based conditions as syringomyelia, or arachnoid cysts, tumor or epidural lipomatosis may also be associated, although not as common.[7]

Cervical radiculopathy in our patient is caused by nerve root compression leading to nerve root distortion, intraneural edema, and focal nerve ischemia. This leads to a localized inflammatory response, chemical mediators within the disc stimulate production of inflammatory cytokines, substance P, bradykinin, tumor necrosis factor alpha, and prostaglandins.[8,9] The membrane surrounding the dorsal root ganglion becomes more permeable, allowing a local inflammatory response that further contributes to radiculopathy.[10] The most common cause of cervical radiculopathy leading to compression is herniated disc. The disc materials are extruded from its normal space and impinge upon the exiting nerve root posterolaterally or intraforaminally.[9]

Degeneration of spine components, that is, osteophytes, facet joint hypertrophy, and ligament hypertrophy,[8,11] can cause decrease in disc height, leading to a "hard disc" bulging with compressive elements.

As far as location, anterior causes (soft or hard disc herniation) and osteophytes from uncinate process are most common causes of radicular symptoms compared with ischemia, trauma, postradiation therapy, neoplasia, and spinal infectious congenital disorders.[11]

Cervical myeloradiculopathy can occur during chronic spondylosis and repetitive compressive changes to the cervical spinal cord and roots and also acutely as a result of flexion and extension injuries.[1,12]

Anterior spondylitic spurs and posterior unfolding ligaments[13] can cause chronic compressive changes and lead to demyelination, vascular compromise, and inflammation of nerve roots.

CLINICAL SIGNS AND SYMPTOMS OF RADICULOPATHY

Neurological symptoms consists of pain, motor weakness and sensory deficits, and reflexes changes (Table 1.1).[9,14] Depending on the nerve root, concurrent symptoms occur in the neck, shoulder, upper arm, and forearm. Pain can vary from dull ache to severe burning. Pain may not be localized because of overlap from multiple roots.[15]

The following patterns of weakness emerge depending on the involved root. Scapular weakness is seen with C4 involvement. Shoulder abduction or forearm flexion weakness with C5;

TABLE 1-1 ■ Nerve Root Levels, Peripheral Nerves, and Muscles of the Upper Limb Commonly Evaluated in the Patient with Neck Pain

Nerve Root Level	Nerve	Muscle
C5, C6	Axillary	Deltoid
C5, C6	Musculocutaneous	Biceps brachii
C5, C6	Suprascapular	Supraspinatus
	Suprascapular	Infraspinatus
C7	Radial	Triceps
	Median	Pronator teres
C8,T1	Median	Abductor pollicis brevis
	Ulnar	First dorsal interossei

From M.J. DePalma, J.J. Gasper, C.W. Slipman, Common neck problems, In: D. Cifu, Braddom's Physical Medicine and Rehabilitation, 5e, Elsevier, St Louis, 2016, p697.

wrist extension, supination with C6; triceps, wrist flexion, and pronation with C7; finger flexion, interosseous weakness with C8 and T1.[16]

If radiculopathy becomes advanced, muscle wasting and fasciculation can be seen.[13]

C7 radiculopathy can produce triceps weakness in 37% and biceps weakness in 28% of patients.[17]

Sensory Changes

C4 nerve root leads to sensory disturbances in shoulder and upper arm, C5 root distribution is lateral arm and thumb.

C6 root leads to changes in lateral forearm and index finger, C7 root to dorsal lateral forearm and third digit. C8 root leads to medial forearm, hand, fourth and fifth digits.[18]

DEEP TENDON REFLEXES

Deep tendon reflexes are muscle stretch reflexes and involuntary responses and can offer an objective assessment for neurologic impairment.[7] In 70% of cases, loss of deep tendon reflexes is the most reliable clinical finding[19] and follows a predictable radicular pattern. In LMN lesions, these reflexes are diminished or lost completely. In UMN lesions, they become exacerbated because of lack of inhibition from central nervous system (CNS).

ELECTROMYOGRAPHY

The electromyography can be used to differentiate cervical radiculopathy from other peripheral nerve involvement, such as peripheral neuropathy and focal nerve entrapment (e.g., carpal tunnel syndrome, ulnar neuropathy), and from cervical myelopathy. If there is involvement of cervical nerve root, leading to nerve damage, denervation potentials (fibrillation potentials and positive sharp waves) can be seen in muscles innervated by that specific nerve root as described earlier.

EMG can further help to prognosticate. If the denervation is severe, then the motor units in that muscle are severely diminished, which indicates poor prognosis. Firing pattern may become rapid with late recruitment. As the nerve root recovers and regeneration begins, polyphasic motor units appear indicating good prognosis.

IMAGING STUDIES

Plain films are very useful in identifying stenosis and degenerative joint disease.[20] According to Brown et al.,[20] anterior-posterior diameter of 13 mm width or less is considered a risk factor for developing myelopathy.

MRI is the best imaging method for evaluating C-spine with high levels of sensitivity (79%–95%) and specificity (82%–88%) for myelopathy. HNP and spondylosis related structural changes are well demonstrated on MRI.[21]

However, the extent of root compression and assessment of functional evaluation is not in the scope of MRI. A soft from a hard disc is difficult to differentiate.[9] Specificity of MRI for nerve root compression is questionable. In one study, 10% of subjects aged younger than 40 years have been noted to have disc herniation. In subjects aged older than 40 years, 20% had evidence of foraminal stenosis and 80% had disc herniation.[22] Therefore MRI should be used in conjunction with history and clinical examination. Computed tomography (CT) is less commonly used in the assessment of degeneration of C-spine. It is limited in its capacity to evaluate soft tissues. A better use of CT is for evaluation of bones for fractures[23] (Fig. 1.2).

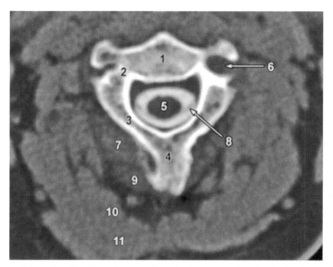

Fig. 1.2 Imaging painful spine disorders. (From L. Czervionke, F. Douglas. Cervical Spine Anatomy. Imaging Painful Spine Disorders, Saunders, Philadelphia, 2011, Fig. 1.3.)

DISCUSSION

Two distinctive elements of differential diagnosis should be considered. One must rule out infectious conditions, such as discitis osteomyelitis, epidural abscess in an intravenous (IV) drug user. Red flags such as fever, chills, history of cancer should be considered.

Other conditions as ALS, multiple sclerosis (MS), and tumors should be ruled out. To do so, an appropriate diagnostic workup should be conducted to narrow the diagnosis.

Prognosis depends upon the level of compression. Although there is limited research available, most authors agree that in most patients nonoperative treatment is effective. In a 1-year cohort study of 26 patients with documented HNP, nonoperative treatment was successful in 92%.[24] A multimodal approach is highly advocated consisting of physical therapy (PT), pharmacotherapy, and surgical referral when necessary.

ACUTE PHASE

Physical Therapy

In the inflammatory phase a short course of cervical immobilization in a soft collar may be beneficial. In some, home cervical traction may decrease symptoms and should be used when acute pain has subsided.[25]

Traction distracts the neural foramen and this decompresses the nerve root. Typically 10 to 12 lbs of traction is applied at 24-degree angle for 20 minutes. There is no sufficient evidence available to prove its efficiency in chronic patients. It is more beneficial when acute pain has subsided and is contraindicated in myelopathy.[26]

Pharmacotherapy

A wide variety of pharmacotherapeutic agents are available. Nonsteroidal antiinflammatory drugs (NSAIDs) have been shown to be effective to alleviate pain and are considered first-line agents. Opioids may be effective for neuropathic pain.[27]

Narcotic analgesics, muscle relaxants, antidepressants, and anticonvulsants are also beneficial in some cases. Tramadol may also prove beneficial in neuropathic pain syndromes,[27] and oral steroids are widely used to treat acute radicular pain via dose packs but no high-quality evidence is available. In view of potential for serious complications, long-term use should be avoided.

SUBACUTE PHASE

After 6 to 8 weeks have passed, subacute phase starts.

Physical Therapy and Manipulation

A monitored, graduated physical therapy program to restore ROM, overall conditioning of neck muscles should be considered. In the first 6 weeks, gentle ROM of neck stretching exercises, supplemented by modalities, including heat, electrical stimulation, and ultrasound is used. Gradual strengthening program follows once pain relief is achieved. There is limited evidence to suggest that manipulation provides short-term benefit in relieving neck pain and cervicogenic headaches.[28]

Steroid Injections

Translaminar, transforaminal epidurals, and nerve root blocks under radiographic guidance are in wide practice currently. These approaches have the advantage of directly infusing the nerve with steroids. One study demonstrated significant pain relief at 14 days and at 6 months,[29] and complications are rare at 1.66%.[30]

CHRONIC PHASE

Referral to Surgery

If a patient fails to respond to nonoperative therapy after a 6-week period, motor weakness is persisting for more than 6 weeks, neurologic deficit is progressive, or the patient develops signs/symptoms of cervical myelopathy, then a referral to the surgeon for intervention is warranted.[31] Surgical referral should not be delayed if there is rapid progression of weakness or development of myelopathy.

Summary

A patient presents with chronic neck pain worsening over time, has neurologic symptoms (weakness, numbness, and pain) along with demonstrable clinical signs of muscle weakness, sensory and reflex changes. The patient was referred to EMG and MRI, which confirmed the diagnosis of cervical radiculopathy in C5–C6 and C6–C7 distribution. Subsequently she received pain management with NSAIDs, muscle relaxants, and a short course of steroid Pac, followed by a 6-week course of PT consisting of cervical traction, stretching modalities, and strengthening. She responded very well. At a follow-up visit 3 months later, patient remained pain free and improved in muscle strengthening by one grade. She uses an occasional Tylenol and continues to remain on home exercise program.

Key Points

- Patients with neck pain should be carefully assessed because the etiology can be diverse and complex.
- Careful attention should be placed to all elements of history and examination.
- Treatment options should be tailored to individual patients.

References

1. J.P. Lewis, R. Rue, R. Byrne, et al., Cervical syrinx as a cause of shoulder pain in 2 athletes, Am. J. Sports Med. 36 (1) (2008) 169–172.
2. I. Thongtrangan, H. Le, J. Park, D.H. Kim, Cauda equina syndrome in patients with low lumbar fractures, Neurosurg. Focus 16 (6) (2004) e6.
3. H. Baba, Y. Maezawa, K. Uchida, et al., Cervical myeloradiculopathy with entrapment neuropathy: a study based on the double crush, Spinal Cord 36 (6) (1998) 399–404.
4. H. Pope, M. Szpalski, R. Gunzburg (Eds.), Cervical Spine Biomechanics. The Degenerative Cervical Spine, Lippincott Williams & Wilkins, Philadelphia, 2001.
5. D.W. Wilson, R.T. Pezzuti, J.N. Place, Magnetic resonance imaging in the preoperative evaluation of cervical radiculopathy, Neurosurgery 28 (2) (1991) 175–179.
6. T.M. Wong, H.B. Leung, W.C. Wong, Correlation between magnetic resonance imaging and radiographic measurement of cervical spine in cervical myelopathy patients, J. Orthop. Surg. (Hong Kong) 12 (2) (2004) 239–242.
7. D.H. Durrant, J.M. True, Myelopathy, Radiculopathy, and Peripheral Entrapment Syndromes, CRC, London, 2002.
8. T.J. Albert, S.E. Murrell, Surgical management of cervical radiculopathy, J. Am. Acad. Orthop. Surg. 7 (6) (1999) 368–376.
9. J.M. Rhee, T. Yoon, K.D. Riew, Cervical radiculopathy, J. Am. Acad. Orthop. Surg. 15 (8) (2007) 485–494.
10. S. Rao, M.G. Fehlings, The optimal radiologic method of assessing spinal cord compromise and cord compression in patients with cervical spinal cord injury: part 1: an evidence based analysis of the published literature, Spine 24 (6) (1999) 598–604.
11. E. Truumees, H.N. Herkowitz, Cervical spondylitic myelopathy and radiculopathy, Instr. Course Lect. 49 (2000) 339–360.
12. S. Ito, M.M. Panjabi, P.C. Ivancic, et al., Spinal canal narrowing during simulated whiplash, Spine 29 (12) (2004) 1330–1339.
13. E. Frank, Approaches to myeloradiculopathy, West. J. Med. 158 (1) (1993) 71–72.
14. D.W. Polston, Cervical radiculopathy, Neurol. Clin. 25 (2) (2007) 373–385.
15. M.R. Ellenberg, J.C. Honet, W.J. Treanor, Cervical radiculopathy, Arch. Phys. Med. Rehabil. 75 (3) (1994) 342–352.
16. Tsao BE, Levin KH, Bodner RA. Comparison of surgical and electrodiagnostic findings in single root lumbosacral radiculopathies. Muscle Nerve. 27 (1) 60–64.
17. C.M. Henderson, R.H. Hennessy, H.M. Shuez, et al., Posterior-lateral foraminotomy as an exclusive operative technique for cervical radiculopathy: a review of 846 consecutively operated cases, Neurosurgery 13 (5) (1983) 504–512.
18. A. Chien, E. Eliav, M. Sterling, Whiplash (grade II) and cervical radiculopathy share a similar sensory presentation: an investigation using quantitative sensory testing, Clin. J. Pain 24 (7) (2008) 595–603.
19. G.L. Marshall, J.W. Little, Deep tendon reflexes: a study of quantitative methods, J. Spinal Cord Med. 25 (2) (2002) 94–99.
20. S. Brown, R. Guthmann, K. Hitchcock, et al., Clinical inquiries: which treatments are effective for cervical radiculopathy? J. Fam. Pract. 58 (2) (2009) 97–99.
21. J.T. Wilmink, Cervical imaging: dynamic aspects and clinical significance, In: M. Szpalski, R. Gunzburg (Eds.), The Degenerative Cervical Spine, Lippincott Williams & Wilkins, Philadelphia, 2001.
22. S.D. Boden, P.R. McCowin, D.O. Davis, et al., Abnormal magnetic-resonance scans of the cervical spine in asymptomatic subjects: a prospective investigation, J. Bone Joint Surg. Am. 72 (8) (1990) 1178–1184.
23. J.Y. Maigne, L. Deligne, Computed tomographic follow-up study of 21 cases of non-operatively treated cervical intervertebral soft disc herniation, Spine 19 (2) (1994) 189–191.
24. J.S. Saal, J.A. Saal, E.F. Yurth, Non-operative management of herniated cervical intervertebral disc with radiculopathy, Spine 21 (16) (1996) 1877–1883.
25. R.L. Swezey, A.M. Swezey, L. Warner, Efficacy of home cervical traction therapy, Am. J. Phys. Med. Rehabil. 78 (1) (1999) 30–32.
26. M.J. Levine, T.J. Acbert, M.D. Smith, Cervical radiculopathy: diagnosis and non-operative management, J. Am. Acad. Orthop. Surg. (4) (1996) 305–316.

27. R.A. Deyo, Drug therapy for back pain which drugs help which patients, Spine 21 (24) (1996) 2840–2849.
28. D.G. Malone, N.G. Baldwin, F.J. Tomecek, et al., Complications of cervical spine manipulation therapy, a 5 year retrospective study in a single group practice, Neurosurg. Focus 13 (6) (2002) ecp1.
29. J.N. Valle, A. Feydy, R.Y. Cartier, et al., Chronic cervical radiculopathy; lateral approach, peri radicular corticosteroid injection, Radiology 218 (3) (2001) 886–892.
30. D.J. Ma, L.A. Gilula, K.D. Riew, Complications of fluoroscopy guided extra-foraminal cervical nerve root blocks an analysis of 1036 injections, J. Bone Joint Surg. Am. 87 (5) (2005) 1025–1030.
31. T.J. Albert, S.E. Murell, Surgical management of cervical radiculopathy, J. Am. Acad. Orthop. Surg. 7 (6) (1999) 368–376.
32. J. Eubanks, Cervical radiculopathy: non-operative management of neck pain and radicular symptoms, J. Am. Fam. Phys. 81 (1) (2010) 33–40.

CHAPTER 2

Back Pain

Dr. Vivek Nagar, MD, MBA ▪ Dr. Michelle Stern, MD

Case Presentation

A 48-year-old obese man presents to the Physical Medicine and Rehabilitation (PM&R) clinic with new onset low back pain. He reports that low back pain, for years without clear onset that intermittently radiates into his right and left posterior thighs, is worse when standing and is associated with morning stiffness. However, he states that he had a sudden onset of back pain 3 weeks ago when he was moving furniture in his home. His pain is located at the lower back and radiates through his left leg. He characterizes his low back pain as cramping and aching and characterizes his left leg pain as burning and electric. His leg pain is worse with sitting and his back pain is worse when coughing. He takes an occasional Tylenol, which seems to help but only temporarily.

REVIEW OF SYSTEMS

He reports associated numbness at the plantar aspect of the left foot. He denies weakness. He denies bowel and bladder incontinence. He denies any weight loss, night sweats, or fevers.

Past medical history: He has a history of hypertension (HTN) for which he is taking Losartan 25 mg daily for the past 10 years.

Social history: Works as a lawyer, recently unemployed 6 months ago. He lives with his wife and two children on the fourth floor with an elevator. He ambulates without assistive device and is independent in his activities of daily living. He smokes 1 pack of cigarettes per day for the past 20 years. He does not drink alcohol or use intravenous drugs.

Allergies: No drug or environmental allergies

Medications: Losartan 25 mg daily, Tylenol as needed

BP: 140/70 mmHg, RR: 16/min, PR: 80 per min, Temp: 97° F, Ht: 5'6", Wt: 220 lbs, BMI 35 kg/m^2

Head, eyes, ear, nose, and throat (HEENT)-extraocular movements (EOMs) full, no ptosis

PHYSICAL EXAMINATION

General: He is alert and oriented. He is in moderate distress because of left-sided back pain.

MUSCULOSKELETAL AND NEUROLOGIC EXAMINATION:

Lateral bending and extension is limited by pain, flexion of trunk is significantly limited by pain

Diffusely rigid and tender to palpation along middle and lower paraspinal muscles

Motor examinaton: right and left lower extremities 5/5

Bilateral Achilles tendon reflex and bilateral patella tendon reflex 2+. Plantar reflex is down-going bilaterally. No clonus bilaterally.

Sensory examination: Dull to light touch along the left lateral thigh, lateral calf, and dorsum of foot. Normal sensation along right lower extremity.

Straight leg test is positive on the left side and negative on the right side

Gait is normal

General Discussion

The approach to a patient with lower back pain (LBP) generally involves categorizing distinct sources of back pain: axial, radicular, and referred pain.[1] Axial lumbosacral pain involves the lumbar region, L1–L5 vertebral segments, and sacral region, S1 to sacrococcygeal region.[1] Axial back pain is commonly used to describe LBP associated with degenerative disc disease without compromise of neural elements. Radicular pain involves radiation of pain that travels through the

TABLE 2.1 ■ **Red Flags**

Trauma
- Major trauma
- Minor trauma in elderly or osteoporotic patients

Infection/Tumor
- History of malignancy
- New onset back pain age <20 years or age <50 years
- Constitutional symptoms
- Recent infection
- Immunosuppression
- Intravenous drug use
- Pain worse at night

Neurologic compromise
- Severe or worsening sensory or motor deficits
- New bowel or bladder dysfunction
- Saddle anesthesia

leg along a dermatomal distribution consistent with a nerve root, or dorsal root ganglion, level compromise, most commonly secondary to mechanical compression. Referred back pain involves pain that travels from a source in a nondermatomal distribution along elements of the same mesodermal origins. Although these terms attempt to simplify etiologies of LBP, LBP is largely a multifactorial condition, including multiple physiologic and psychosocial factors that remain difficult to define, diagnose, and treat.[1]

Once categorized, the determination of potentially progressive or unstable etiology of back pain is paramount (Table 2.1). "Red flags" are used to determine such etiologies, including cancer, infection, trauma, and neurologic compromise. These findings include fevers/night sweats/chills, bowel or bladder incontinence, "saddle anesthesia" (decreased sensation around the perineum, groin, and/or medial thighs), thoracic pain, gait ataxia, or prior history of cancer or high impact trauma. Positive findings should prompt emergent evaluation, either via imaging and/or referral to specialists (surgery, oncology, etc.).

As with any evaluation, a thorough history and physical examination are essential in diagnosis of lumbosacral radiculopathy. Regarding history, a complete description of pain is necessary, including onset, location, duration, characterization, alleviating and aggravating factors, radiation, timing, and severity. Associated paresthesias, such as numbness, tingling, and weakness, can often be appreciated as well. Of significant importance is associating these symptoms to a specific dermatomal and/or myotomal level for radicular back pain, requiring focal questioning (Fig. 2.1). Regarding physical examination, a comprehensive neurologic examination is necessary, including assessment of motor strength and evaluation for upper motor findings (Fig. 2.2). In addition, certain special maneuvers can guide to specific etiologies of low back pain as discussed earlier, such as facet loading test (axial back pain, facet arthropathy), straight leg raise and Slump test with reproduction of symptoms (radicular back pain, L4 to S1 radiculopathy), reverse straight leg raise, and Ely test with reproduction of symptoms (radicular back pain, –L4 radiculopathy; Table 2.2).

Differential Diagnosis

1. **Myofascial pain**—most commonly localized to the low back. There may be radiation to the bilateral lower extremities along the posterior buttocks and thighs. This referral of pain is not consistent with a dermatomal distribution, and should not be mistaken for radiculopathy.[2]

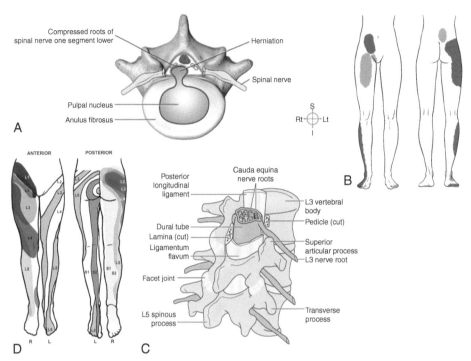

Fig. 2.1 Lumbar radiculopathy. (With permission from: (A) B. Liebgott, The Anatomical Basis of Dentistry, 4e, Mosby, Elsevier, 2017; (B) C.C. Goodman, J. Heick, R.T. Lazaro, Differential Diagnosis for Physical Therapists: Screening for Referral, 6e, Saunders, Elsevier, 2017; (C) W.R. Frontera, T.D. Rizzo, J.K. Silver, Essentials of Physical Medicine and Rehabilitation: Musculoskeletal Disorders, Pain, and Rehabilitation, 4e, Elsevier, 2018; (D) W.S. Bartynski, K.A. Petropoulou, The MR imaging features and clinical correlates in low back pain related syndromes. Magn. Res. Imaging Clin. N. Am. 15 (2007) 137–154.)

2. **Degenerative spine disease**
   Discogenic pain: Most commonly associated with low back pain worse with flexion, sitting, twisting, and increased abdominal pressure (coughing, sneezing).[3]
   Facet arthropathy: Most commonly associated with extension and lateral bending. Classically associated with facet-loading test positive; however, studies have shown it is unreliable in diagnosing facet arthropathy mediated pain alone.[4]
3. **Lumbosacral radiculopathy**—most commonly associated with leg pain, oftentimes will supersede lumbar pain, such that patients will experience leg pain greater than back pain.[5] This pain usually radiates in a dermatomal fashion, associated with the pathologic nerve root.
4. **Lumbar stenosis**—can present with low back pain, neurogenic claudication (discomfort, pain, numbness or weakness in the calves, buttocks, or thighs that is precipitated in lumbar extension and relieved in lumbar flexion), sensory disturbances in dermatomal and nondermatomal fashion, motor weakness, and pathologic reflexes.[6]
5. **Lumbar postlaminectomy syndrome**—commonly described as "failed back surgery syndrome"; it is defined by International Association for the Study of Pain as "lumbar spinal pain of unknown origin either persisting despite surgical intervention or appearing after surgical intervention for spinal pain originally in the same topographic location."[7] Comprehensive history should include evaluation of preoperative risk factors (psychosocial factors, smoking, obesity), intraoperative risk factors (operating at a single level, operating at the wrong level), and postoperative risk factors.[8]

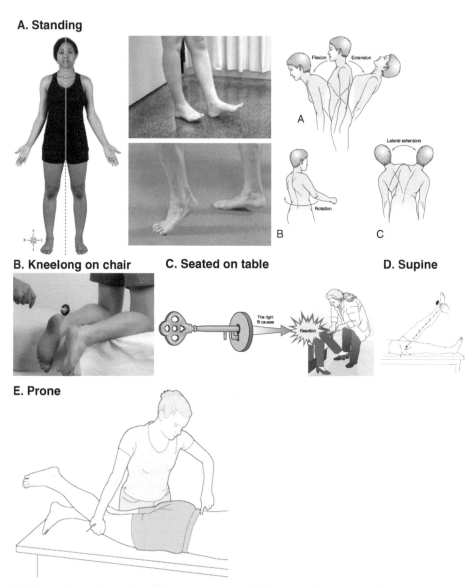

Fig. 2.2 Lumbar radiculopathy. (With permission from: (A) K. Patton, G. Thibodeau, Structure & Function of the Body, 16e, Elsevier, St Louis, 2020, Fig. 1-3; T. Cueco, Essential Guide to the Cervical Spine: Volume One: Clinical Assessment and Therapeutic Approaches, Elsevier, Philadelphia, 2016, Fig. 8-63; R.C. Evans, Illustrated Orthopedic Physical Assessment, 3e, Mosby, Philadelphia, 2009, Fig. 8-77; M.H. Swartz, Textbook of Physical Diagnosis: History and Examination, 8e, Elsevier, Philadelphia, 2021, Fig. 20-22; (B) N.J. Talley, S. O'Connor. Clinical Examination Volume One: A SysGuide to Physical Diagnosis, 8e, 2018, Fig. 28-11; (C) A. Guerra, K. Davis, Mosby's Pharmacy Technician: Principles and Practice, 5e, Churchill Livingstone, Australia, 2019, Fig. 17-5; (D) V.J. Devlin, Spine Secrets, 3e, Elsevier, Philadelphia, 2021, Fig. 1-3; (E) L. Chaitow, J. DeLany, Clinical Application of Neuromuscular Techniques: Volume 2: The Lower Body, 2e, Churchill Livingstone, London, 2012, Fig. 10-39.)

TABLE 2.2 ■ Diagnosis of Lumbar Radiculopathy

Nerve Root	Pain Radiation	Gait Deviation	Motor Weakness	Sensory Loss	Reflex Loss
L3	Groin and inner thigh	Sometimes antalgic	Hip flexion	Anteromedial thigh	Patellar (variable)
L4	Anterior thigh or knee, or upper medial leg	Sometimes antalgic Difficulty rising onto a stool or chair with one leg	Knee extension, hip flexion and adduction	Lateral or anterior thigh, medial leg, and knee	Patellar
L5	Buttocks, anterior or lateral leg, dorsal foot	Difficulty heel walking; if more severe, then foot slap or steppage gait Trendelenburg gait	Ankle dorsiflexion, foot eversion and inversion, toe extension, hip abduction	Posterolateral thigh, antero-lateral leg, and mid-dorsal foot	Medial hamstring (variable)
S1	Posterior thigh, calf, plantar foot	Difficulty toe walking or cannot rise on toes 20 times	Foot plantar flexion	Posterior thigh and calf, lateral and plantar foot	Achilles

(With permission from M.J. Ellenberg, M. Ellenberg, Lumbar Radiculopathy, In: W.R. Frontera, J.K. Silver, T.D. Rizzo (eds), Essentials of Physical Medicine and Rehabilitation, 4e, Elsevier, 2019, pp257–263.

6. **Other causes of low back pain:**
   a. Cauda equina syndrome: Constellation of symptoms indicating neurologic compromise related to dysfunction of the ropelike nerve fibers at the distal spinal cord, most commonly caused by large lumbar disc prolapse with compression.[9] These symptoms include, but are not limited to, saddle anesthesia, sexual dysfunction, fecal incontinence, bladder dysfunction, and lower limb weakness. Magnetic resonance imaging (MRI) is the choice of imaging, and treatment is urgent surgical decompression unless medically contraindicated.[9]
   b. Tumor: The strongest risk factor for back pain secondary to bone metastasis is a history of cancer.[10] Those cancers associated with bone metastasis include breast, lung, renal cell, and prostate cancers.[11]
   c. Infection: A comprehensive history of infection related to low back pain includes recent fevers, malaise, spinal injections, epidural catheter placement, intravenous drug use, and immunosuppression.[12]
   d. There are numerous other causes of nonspine-related back pain, including fibromyalgia, piriformis syndrome, hip osteoarthritis, and aortic aneurysm

Case Discussion

Our patient presents with acute on chronic low back pain. In evaluating this patient, it is important to delineate his separate pain complaints. On one hand, he describes insidious onset of low back pain, which suggests chronicity. Given his chronic description of aching pain in the low back without dermatomal radiation, risk factors of obesity and smoking, physical examination findings of paraspinal tenderness and rigidity, this patient likely has axial back pain. Therefore differential diagnoses should include those associated with degenerative spine changes, such as discogenic disease, facet arthritis, and spondylosis.

On the other hand, he describes clear onset of pain after an inciting incident, which suggests acuity. Along with history of pain and numbness along L5 dermatome and physical examination findings of positive straight leg test, this patient likely has lumbosacral radiculopathy as well. Therefore differential diagnoses should include space occupying lesions resulting in compression of the L5 nerve root from the central canal to the neural foramen, including disc herniation, degenerative spondylosis, neural foraminal stenosis, and fractures.

DIAGNOSTIC TESTING

In the absence of red flags, trauma, prior spinal surgery, and refractory back pain to conservative management, diagnostic testing is not indicated in the majority of patients with low back pain. Initial treatment should be geared toward conservative management.[13]

Presently, there is no one type of imaging that shows a clear advantage over others. X-rays are a simple, cost-effective method of evaluation of bony anatomy to reveal gross bony abnormalities commonly associated with degenerative spine disease (such as disc space narrowing, osteophyte formation, neuroforaminal stenosis, facet arthropathy), misalignment (spondylolisthesis), and trauma (vertebral fractures, pars interarticularis fractures). X-rays are commonly used for chronic, persistent low back pain with acute pain associated with new red flags secondary to trauma, including fracture or instability. Flexion and extension views are recommended to evaluate symptomatic spondylolisthesis.[5]

In patients with refractory radicular pain syndrome (radicular low back pain lasting 4–6 weeks after conservative management), MRI is considered the gold standard for imaging given its sensitivity for soft tissue evaluation, including disc, tumor, muscle, and nerve involvement. Of note, it is important to evaluate MRI with a high pretest probability, garnered from a precise clinical suspicion based on history and physical examination. Lumbosacral MRI examinations are more likely to be "abnormal" by age 40 years in asymptomatic individuals, and herniated discs are not infrequently found in asymptomatic young adults.[5]

For patients who cannot undergo MRI, computed tomography (CT) remains an alternative option. Although routine CT is not recommended for acute, subacute, or chronic nonspecific or radicular low back pain, CT is recommended for patients with refractory radicular pain who are in consideration for epidural steroid injections. If these patients are in consideration for surgical discectomy or have a history of prior spinal surgery with hardware, CT myelography is recommended.

Bone scans can be used to evaluate for osteomyelitis, occult fractures, and inflammatory arthropathy. Single-photon emission CT (SPECT) imaging has also been used to evaluate inflammatory arthropathy, specifically that of the sacroiliac (SI) joint; however, SPECT imaging is not currently recommended for low back pain evaluation.[5] Although discography, when paired with MRI or CT, can provide anatomic information for surgical decisions regarding discectomy for significant radiculopathy, the lack of standardization in discography leads to low predictive value and is currently moderately not recommended for evaluation of acute, subacute, and chronic low back and radicular pain.[14]

Electrodiagnostic studies (EDX), primarily electromyography (EMG), can be used to evaluate radicular pain syndromes. It can be useful to determine if neurologic compromise is present, chronicity of symptoms, and/or aggravation of preexisting injury.[15] However, it is important to note that EDX tests only motor axonal loss or conduction block, and would not yield abnormalities affecting the sensory nerve root. Therefore EDX is not recommended for low back pain without radicular pain symptoms. In addition, EMG represents a high specificity, low sensitivity test for radiculopathy, serving as a good way to confirmatory test rather than a screening test. Therefore it is important to use EDX studies as a supplement to clinical decision making and EDX results are interpreted in the realm of prevalence of suspected pathology.[16]

Case Discussion

Our patient presents with radicular low back pain syndrome. Although he has not completed any conservative management, he does have a history of an inciting, traumatic event. Therefore imaging with X-rays would not be unreasonable.

Because our patient does not exhibit constitutional symptoms, neurologic compromise on examination, or red flags, further diagnostic testing is not indicated. Although MRI would not be necessary at this time, it could yield important information regarding further treatment options, such as interventional management.

Objective Data

X-ray lumbosacral spine—mild lumbar disc space narrowing suggested at L3–S1 without significant change in position of vertebral bodies in alignment upon flexion and extension. Mild diffuse spondylosis is seen without visualized compression fracture. Mild to moderate facet arthropathy is noted in the lower lumbar spine. The pedicles and vertebral heights are intact. The SI joints are patent and symmetric bilaterally.

MRI lumbar spine without contrast—degenerative changes and diffuse ligamentum flavum hypertrophy throughout causing mild to moderate spinal stenosis and mild bilateral neural foraminal stenosis at L3 through S1. Most pronounced, left sided L4–L5 posterolateral disc protrusion.

Laboratory work—complete blood count (CBC) within normal limits. Erythrocyte sedimentation rate (ESR) and C-reactive protein (CRP) within normal limits.

On comprehensive review of our patient, he presents with acute L5 radiculopathy on chronic axial low back pain. Regarding his axial back pain, imaging reveals multiple possible etiologies, including degenerative discs, facet arthropathy, and spondylosis. Given his history of pain with extension and morning stiffness, his axial back pain is likely related to facet arthropathy. Regarding his radicular pain, imaging reveals two possible etiologies, including disc herniation and neural foraminal stenosis. Although both processes could cause radiculopathy, the acuity of his presentation suggests that disc herniation is the likely etiology. Diffuse neural foraminal stenosis is likely the result of ongoing degenerative spine disease, and is likely not the primary etiology of his radiculopathy.

Review of Proposed Pathology and Pathobiomechanics

The majority of back pain is caused by myofascial low back pain, which is usually caused by back sprain or lumbago. Myofascial pain is likely a result of stress applied to muscle or ligament resulting from primary trauma or secondary continuous postural instability. Myofascial pain may be associated with trigger points, defined as taut muscle bands secondary to chronic contractions.[2]

The most widely accepted theory of degenerative spine disease is described in a three-phase model:[17]

Phase 1: Dysfunctional phase, characterized by repetitive microtrauma causing annular fissures and tears in the disc, leading to predispositions to disc herniation, inability to retain water, and loss of disc height

Phase 2: Instability phase, characterized by progressive disc tears and disc height loss, leading to additional mechanical stress on the facet joints

Phase 3: Stabilization phase, characterized by further disc height narrowing, fibrosis, and osteophyte formation

This degeneration of the disc cascades stress-induced osteophyte formation throughout the lumbosacral spine is known as spondylosis. Areas of the spine that are commonly associated with degenerative changes include the facet joints and sacroiliac joints. Degenerative changes in the facet joint, also known as facet arthropathy, can also be seen with paraspinal muscle rigidity and weakness. Spondylosis results in osteophyte production that can become either primary pain generators in axial back pain or secondary pain generators in radicular back pain caused by compression on neural elements. Lumbosacral radiculopathy or stenosis is described as a condition in which the spinal cord and nerve roots are entrapped in one of three anatomic locations: (1) central canal, (2) neural foramen, (3) lateral recess. Etiologies of central canal and neuroforaminal stenosis include disc herniation, ligamentum flavum hypertrophy, articular facet hypertrophy, posterior longitudinal ligament ossification, and vertebral body subluxation (spondylolisthesis).[18] Lumbar radiculopathy is most commonly caused by lesions of discs and

---

TABLE 2.3 ■ General Physical Therapy Program for Low Back

Lumbar stabilization:
1. Local segmental stability: pelvic tilting exercises (most commonly accentuating posterior pelvic tilt to decrease mechanical stress on lumbar spine), core stabilization exercises (strengthening abdominal wall)
2. Closed chain stability exercises: focus on strengthening weight-bearing muscles with gravity-dependent stretch (gluteus maximus/gluteus medius/abdominal wall) with squats, balance board
3. Open chain stability exercises: assisted stretching and strengthening of specific muscles as necessary to assist proper closed chain stability exercises (hip flexor stretch, such as iliopsoas and quadriceps, hamstring stretch, or gluteus medius strengthening)

---

degenerative disease of the spine. Most incidences are self-limiting and resolve within 1 to 2 weeks (50% of cases) or 6 to 12 weeks (90% of cases).[13] Lumbar radiculopathy and lumbar stenosis share similar pathologic mechanisms with regard to mechanical compression. Another theory regarding lumbar stenosis is that of vascular compression, a compression of local vascular structures that leads to transient ischemia of the spinal cord from arterial insufficiency and venous stasis.

Treatment Strategies

Low back pain treatment depends on its etiologies, presence of radiculopathy, and physical or radiologic findings.[19] Based on general consensus, conservative management is considered first-line management. Conservative management consists of multiple modalities, including physical and rehabilitation therapy, pharmacologic treatment, psychological treatment, and complementary and alternative medicine approaches.[1]

Physical therapy has been shown to have a greater improvement on acute low back pain than chronic low back pain. Stretching exercise is most associated with pain reduction, whereas strengthening exercise is most associated with functional gains.[1] Strengthening exercise is aimed toward the multifidus muscles, transverse abdominis muscles, and deep muscles of the spine that aid in lumbar stability. Lumbar stabilization is commonly used for disc herniation treatment to improve proprioceptive senses of the tissues in surrounding joints.[20] Early enrollment of physical therapy in acute low back pain leads to decreased health services utilization and improved pain outcomes compared with late physical therapy.[21]

McKenzie method is a widely accepted physiotherapy technique for low back pain, based on the premise of correlating patient preference in directional movement with exercise prescription to decrease pain. McKenzie method is assumed to be an extension-based therapy, but it is meant to be a highly individualized prescription based on specific patients. However, there is still little efficacy for use of McKenzie method for chronic low back pain.[22]

Multidisciplinary therapy (physical and psychological therapy combined), acupuncture, massage, and spinal manipulation have small to moderate effects on pain and function in chronic, nonradicular low back pain. Although many other modalities are commonly used in practice, such as ultrasound, electrical nerve stimulation, lumbar supports, and taping, a lack of randomized control trials lead to inadequate data to confirm benefit of use in low back pain.

See Table 2.3 for general low back physical therapy program protocol.

Pharmacologic treatments are fundamental in acute and chronic low back treatments. Acetaminophen and nonsteroidal antiinflammatory drugs (NSAIDs) are commonly prescribed medications, which are effective in short-term pain relief. Acetaminophen is generally preferred given its safer side-effect profile. When selecting NSAIDs, use of the lowest effective dose for the

TABLE 2.4 ■ Differential Diagnosis, Physical Examination, Physical Therapy Program, Interventions

	Pain Description	Physical Examination	Physical Therapy Program	Interventions
Myofascial	Pain worse at end range of motion, with possible radiation to posterior thighs	Diffuse pain with palpation, ± trigger points	Massage, initial stretching phase followed by strengthening phase	Trigger point injections
Facet-mediated	Pain worse with extension, associated with stiffness	Facet-loading positive, pain with lateral bending	Williams flexion-based therapy	Medial branch nerve blocks and ablation, Facet joint injections
Discogenic	Pain worse with flexion, without radiation, pain with Valsalva	Pain with forward flexion	McKenzie extension-based therapy	Disc biacuplasty, IDET
Disc herniation	Pain that radiates to lower extremities in dermatomal distribution, pain with Valsalva	Straight leg positive, Slump test positive	Posterolateral herniation: extension-based therapy Far lateral herniation: flexion-based therapy	Transforaminal epidural steroid injection, discectomy
Spondylolisthesis	Pain worse with movement, improved at rest	Pain with flexion or extension	Lumbar stabilization therapy	Bracing, surgery if needed
Sacroiliac Joint	Inferior low back/buttock pain, worse with sitting, intermittent radiation to the posterior thighs	FABER positive, SI distraction	General low back program	Sacroiliac joint steroid injection
Lumbar stenosis	Pain with intermittent radiation into posterior thighs or dermatomal distribution, ± neurogenic claudication	Pain with extension, ± Straight leg or Slump test	General low back program	Epidural steroid injection, decompression (minimally invasive vs. traditional)

FABER, Flexion, abduction, external rotation; IDET, intradiscal electrothermal therapy; SI, sacroiliac.

shortest duration is recommended given its renal, cardiovascular, and gastrointestinal side effects. Skeletal muscle relaxants have shown short-term relief for analgesic effects; however, there is limited evidence to definitely show differences in efficacy between them. Side-effect profiles to be considered include central nervous system depression and risk for falls. Tramadol and opioids should only be considered as last-line management for low back pain that is refractory to aforementioned therapies. Although potent opioids have shown significant analgesia, their potential for dependence and tolerance discourages any long-term use.[14]

Interventional management is reserved for patients with refractory low back pain to conservative measures. There are a number of interventional strategies that are targeted toward etiologies of back pain in conjunctional with appropriate conservative management (Table 2.4):

Myofascial pain: trigger point injections

Facet-mediated arthropathy: facet joint injections, medial branch nerve blocks, medial branch nerve ablations[4]

Discogenic: disc biacuplasty, intradiscal electrothermography[23]

Stenosis (central or neural foraminal): transforaminal epidural steroid injection, interlaminar steroid injection[24]

Disc herniation: minimally invasive discectomy, open discectomy[25]

Spondylolisthesis: decompression (laminectomy) and fusion[26]

Summary

This patient presented with acute on chronic low back pain, along with radiating symptoms along a dermatome. Given the nature of traumatic event, this patient underwent imaging with x-ray and MRI of the lumbar spine, which revealed degenerative spondylosis, multilevel neuroforaminal stenosis, and left-sided L4–L5 posterolateral disc protrusion. By pairing this patient's history, physical, and imaging findings, he was diagnosed with acute L5 radiculopathy with underlying lumbar spondylosis. The patient was educated on exercise modifications and was referred to physical therapy. This patient underwent a 6-week physical therapy program that consisted of general low back program along with McKenzie extension-based exercises. His back pain is now manageable, and he is able to go to work. He continues to perform exercises at home as instructed during therapy.

> ### Key Points
>
> - Patients with low back pain must be carefully assessed. Red flags should always be addressed during every encounter.
> - Imaging can help guide therapy, but should not substitute clinical judgment in making a diagnosis.
> - Conservative measures are highly effective if exercises are modified to tailor a specific location of pathology or diagnosis.

References

1. I. Urits, A. Burshtein, M. Sharma, et al., Low back pain, a comprehensive review: pathophysiology, diagnosis, and treatment, Curr. Pain Headache Rep. 23 (2019) 23.

2. A. Tantanatip, K.V. Chang, Pain, myofascial syndrome. [Updated 2019 Jun 18], In: StatPearls [Internet], StatPearls Publishing, Treasure Island (FL), 2019 January. Available from: https://www.ncbi.nlm.nih.gov/books/NBK499882/.

3. T.M. Annaswamy, C. Taylor, Lumbar disc disorders. [Updated 2017 Aug 18], In: PM&R Knowledge Now [Internet], American Academy of Physical Medicine and Rehabilitation, Rosemont (IL), 2020 November.

4. C.E. Alexander, M. Varacallo, Lumbosacral facet syndrome. [Updated 2019 Mar 23], In: StatPearls [Internet], StatPearls Publishing, Treasure Island (FL), 2019 January. Available from: https://www.ncbi.nlm.nih.gov/books/NBK441906/.

5. K. Hegmann, R. Travis, R.M. Belcourt, et al., Diagnostic tests for low back disorders, J. Occup. Environm. Med. 61 (4) (2019) 155–161.

6. A. Raja, S. Hoang, O. Viswanath, et al., Spinal stenosis. [Updated 2020 Apr 28], In: StatPearls [Internet], StatPearls Publishing, Treasure Island (FL), 2020 January. Available from: https://www.ncbi.nlm.nih.gov/books/NBK441989/.

7. Z. Baber, M.A. Erdek, Failed back surgery syndrome: current perspectives, J. Pain Res. 9 (2016) 979–987.

8. V.J. Orhurhu, R. Chu, J. Gill, Failed back surgery syndrome. [Updated 2019 Mar 26], In: StatPearls [Internet], StatPearls Publishing, Treasure Island (FL), 2019 January. Available from: https://www.ncbi.nlm.nih.gov/books/NBK539777/.

9. A. Quaile, Cauda equina syndrome-the questions, Int. Orthopaed. 43 (2019) 957–961.
10. R. Chou, Low back pain, American College of Physicians, Ann. Intern. Med. 160 (2014) ITC6–1.
11. R.A. Deyo, J. Rainville, D.L. Kent, What can the history and physical examination tell us about low back pain? J. Am. Med. Assoc. 268 (1992) 760.
12. R.A. Deyo, J.N. Weinstein, Low back pain, N. Engl. J. Med. 344 (2001) 363–370.
13. C.E. Alexander, M. Varacallo, Lumbosacral radiculopathy. [Updated 2019 mar 23], In: StatPearls [Internet], StatPearls Publishing, Treasure Island (FL), 2019 January. Available from: https://www.ncbi.nlm.nih.gov/books/NBK430837/.
14. K. Fujii, M. Yamazaki, J.D. Kang, et al., Discogenic back pain: literature review of definition, diagnosis, and treatment, JBMR Plus 3 (5) (2019) e10180.
15. P.B. Kang, D.C. Preston, E.M. Raynor, Involvement of superficial peroneal sensory nerve in common peroneal neuropathy, Muscle Nerve 31 (2005) 725–729.
16. K. Barrette, J. Levin, D. Miles, D.J. Kennedy, The value of electrodiagnostic studies in predicting treatment outcomes for patients with spine pathologies, Phys. Med. Rehabil. Clin. North Am. 29 (4) (2018) 681–687.
17. W.H. Kirkaldy-Willis, The pathology and pathogenesis of low back pain, In: Managing Low Back Pain, Churchill Livingstone, New York, NY, 1988, 49.
18. A. Raja, A. Hanna, S. Hoang, et al., Spinal stenosis. [Updated 2019 Jul 13], In: StatPearls [Internet], StatPearls Publishing, Treasure Island (FL), 2019 January. Available from: https://www.ncbi.nlm.nih.gov/books/NBK441989/.
19. H.C. Wenger, A.S. Cifu, Treatment of low back pain, J. Am. Med. Assoc. 318 (2017) 743–744.
20. D.-K. Jeong, Effect of lumbar stabilization exercise on disc herniation index, sacral angle, and functional improvement in patients with lumbar disc herniation, J. Phys. Ther. Sci. 29 (2017) 2121–2125.
21. E. Arnold, J. La Barrie, L. DaSilva, et al., The effect of timing of physical therapy for acute low back pain on health services utilization: a systematic review, Arch. Phys. Med. Rehabil. 100 (2019) 1324–1338.
22. A. Dunsford, S. Kumar, S. Clarke, Integrating evidence into practice: use of McKenzie-based treatment for mechanical low back pain, J. Multidiscip. Healthc. 4 (2011) 393–402.
23. S. Helm Ii, T.T. Simopoulos, M. Stojanovic, S. Abdi, M.A. El Terany, Effectiveness of thermal annular procedures in treating discogenic low back pain, Pain Physician 20 (2017) 447–470.
24. K. Patel, S. Upadhyayula, Epidural steroid injections. [Updated 2019 May 2], In: StatPearls [Internet], StatPearls Publishing, Treasure Island (FL), 2019 January. Available from: https://www.ncbi.nlm.nih.gov/books/NBK470189/.
25. M.R. Rasouli, V. Rahimi-Movaghar, F. Shokraneh, M. Moradi-Lakeh, R. Chou, Minimally invasive discectomy versus microdiscectomy/open discectomy for symptomatic lumbar disc herniation, Cochrane Database Syst. Rev. 9 (2014) CD010328.
26. T.L. Schulte, F. Ringel, M. Quante, et al., Surgery for adult spondylolisthesis: a systematic review of the evidence, Eur. Spine J. 25 (2016) 2539–2567.

CHAPTER 3

Shoulder Pain

Dr. Se Won Lee, MD ▪ Dr. Eric Aguila, MD

Case Presentation

A 50-year-old, right-hand-dominant woman presents to the Physical Medicine and Rehabilitation (PM&R) clinic with a history of left shoulder pain. She describes her pain as aching and sharp. She experiences worsening pain on movement of the shoulder, especially with overhead activities. She reports intermittent mild shoulder pain for many years, but her current symptoms of left shoulder pain have become constant over the past 4 to 5 months. She occasionally takes acetaminophen and ibuprofen, which provides some temporary relief. The pain results in occasional disruption of her sleep. She has not seen any other physician for her symptoms nor had any previous workup.

Past medical history and medications: Hypertension for 6 years and noninsulin-dependent diabetes for the past 4 years and hypercholesterolemia.

Social history: She works as a lawyer, lives with family in a house with 12 steps. She has one 16-year-old daughter.

Past surgical history: None

Allergies: No known drug allergy.

Medications: Lisinopril 40 mg once a day, metformin, 500 mg twice a day, and lovastatin 40 mg at night

BP: 130/70 mmHg, RR: 14/min, PR: 75 per min, Temp: 97° F, Ht: 5'8", Wt: 160 lbs. BMI: 24.3 kg/m^2

PHYSICAL EXAMINATION

Cranial nerves: Extraocular movement (EOM) is full, no ptosis, face symmetric, tongue-midline. Shrugging shoulder: Symmetric

General: Alert, oriented, and in mild distress because of right-sided shoulder pain.

Extremities: No edema, no skin rashes or erythema, no vasomotor instability, no surgical scars. No gross atrophy noted.

NEUROMUSCULOSKELETAL EXAMINATION

Range of motion (ROM) of neck: Full in all directions.

ROM of left shoulder: Abduction: 60 degrees, flexion: 70 degrees, external rotation: 30 degrees. Exaggerated scapular movement on abduction.

ROM of right shoulder: Full in all directions.

Motor examination: Left upper extremity (LUE) all groups 5/5. Right upper extremity (RUE) 2/5 in shoulder abduction and forward flexion with pain.

All other muscles were 5/5.

Deep tendon reflex (DTR): 2+ in biceps, triceps, and brachioradialis.

Sensory examination: Intact to light touch and pinprick sensation in both upper extremities.

Gait was within normal limits without any deviations.

Tone was normal.

Labs: White blood cell (WBC): 6800, cell/mL; hemoglobin (Hg): 12.0 g/dL

HgA1C: 7.1

General Discussion: General Approach to Shoulder Pain

The initial focus when evaluating this patient should attempt to differentiate local shoulder pathologies versus referred/radiating pain from cervical spine pathologies, although coexisting lesions are possible and common. The areas on which to focus in this patient's history involve recognizing significant cervical spine symptoms and focal neurologic deficits, including motor

TABLE 3.1 ■ Regional Musculoskeletal Pain Generators Based on the Location of Pain

Location of Pain	Common Musculoskeletal Disorders
Anterolateral	Subacromial impingement syndrome 　- Subacromial/subdeltoid bursitis: constant shoulder pain and night pain 　- Rotator cuff (supra/infraspinatus) tendinopathy/tear: varying pain with movement
Superior	Acromioclavicular (AC) sprain, degenerative joint disease, distal clavicular osteolysis and osteomyelitis SLAP (superior labral tear from anterior to posterior): often asymptomatic
Anteromedial	Bicipital tendinopathy and biceps tendon subluxation and tear 　- Location of tenderness (on bicipital groove) changes with humeral rotation 　- Subcoracoid impingement syndrome with/without bursitis, subscapularis tendinopathy, and tear 　- Pain/tenderness immediately under/lateral to coracoid process
Medial	Sternoclavicular degenerative joint disease, sprain, subluxation, dislocation, or infection 　- Reproducible pain with cross-arm adduction or end range of abduction
Posterior	Subacromial impingement Internal impingement syndrome Rotator cuff (infraspinatus or teres minor) tendinopathy/tear, calcific tendinopathy Myofascial pain syndrome of rhomboids, trapezius muscles with specific referred pain pattern Scapulothoracic bursitis: aggravated by scapular retraction, shoulder abduction/external rotation Cervical facet arthropathy: spondylosis, trauma (whiplash), worse pain on extension/rotation of cervical spine (nonspecific)
Poorly localized	Adhesive capsulitis (often diffuse, poorly localized), glenohumeral arthritis (osteoarthritis, inflammatory arthropathy), osteonecrosis, glenoid labral tears, and fracture

(From S.W. Lee. Musculoskeletal Injuries and Conditions: Assessment and Management, Demos Medical, New York, 2017.)

and sensory deficit of upper extremities (UE). The mode of onset, the exact location of the pain, aggravating, and relieving factors would be important in establishing a differential diagnosis (Table 3.1). For example, the pain from cervical spine pathologies can be reproducible with cervical spine motion (or movement) rather than shoulder movement. Acute and abrupt onset may suggest trauma or vascular event as the underlying etiology. Rapid development of pain may suggest an inflammatory or infectious process as the underlying etiology.

The presence of sensory or motor deficits in the UEs may implicate neuropathy (cervical root, brachial plexus, mononeuropathy) as the cause of her shoulder pain (Table 3.2). True muscle weakness from neural origin should be differentiated from the weakness caused by musculoskeletal pain or impaired range of motion (ROM).

Physical examination should be geared toward the differential diagnosis based on history taking, including the musculoskeletal examination of cervical and shoulder pathologies and neurologic examination to differentiate neuropathic versus musculoskeletal processes.

Common Differential Diagnoses for Shoulder Pain

1. **Subacromial impingement syndrome**—process involves impingement of structures in the subacromial region between the acromion (coracoacromial arch) and humeral head/neck (particularly, greater tuberosity). The subacromial subdeltoid bursa and supra/infraspinatus tendon are commonly impinged, causing bursitis and tendinopathy and subsequently tear (Fig. 3.1).

TABLE 3.2 ■ **Typical Neuropathic Pain Generators**[26]

Pathology	Characteristics
C5, 6 radiculopathy	Significant neck pain commonly ± sensory and motor deficits in the C5-6 root distribution
Brachial amyotrophy (Parsonage-Turner syndrome)	Typically presents with initial severe pain (≥7/10 on the numeric rating scale) with gradual improvement of pain followed by muscle atrophy and weakness
Suprascapular neuropathy (at suprascapular notch or spinoglenoid fossa)	Present with deep, posterior pain with muscle atrophy (supraspinatus, infraspinatus)
Axillary neuropathy (at quadrilateral space	Present with deep posterior shoulder pain with atrophy (deltoid and teres minor)[27]

Data from [26, 27]

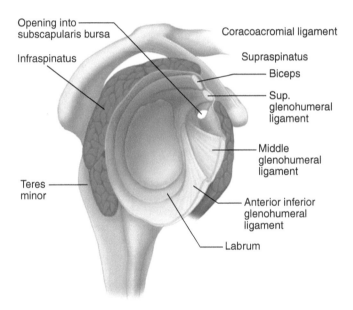

Fig. 3.1 A sagittal view of the glenohumeral joint showing the glenohumeral ligament, glenoid labrum, and biceps tendon. *Sup.*, Superior. (From T.S. Mologne, Shoulder Anatomy and Biomechanics. Delee, Drez, & Miller's Orthopaedic Sports Medicine: Principles and Practice, Elsevier, Philadelphia, 2020, 399–401.)

The pain is located on the anterolateral aspect of the shoulder, beneath the acromion, down to the deltoid tuberosity, typically aggravated by positions or activities to narrow down the subacromial space, such as overhead activities requiring abduction and internal rotation of the humerus (engaging the greater tuberosity under the coracoacromial arch). Although this is the descriptive diagnosis to explain the mechanism, it is frequently used interchangeably with rotator cuff tendinopathy (or syndrome) or subacromial bursitis.

2. **Other shoulder impingement syndromes**—although subacromial impingement syndrome is the most common, there are other shoulder impingement syndromes, including internal impingement syndrome, subcoracoid impingement syndrome, and so on. These conditions

were less well known than subacromial impingement syndrome but illustrate distinctive mechanisms with different presentations. Subcoracoid impingement syndrome is the impingement of subscapularis tendon or subcoracoid/subdeltoid bursa between the lesser tuberosity of humerus and coracoid process. The pain is located in the anterior aspect of the shoulder (rather than anterolateral aspect in subacromial impingement) and provocation maneuver/activity is slightly different with adduction added to flexion and internal rotation of the humerus. Internal impingement is a less well-known cause of posterior shoulder pain. However, it is a relatively common cause of shoulder pain in a specific population (e.g., throwing athletes, such as pitcher, tennis player). The posterior part of supraspinatus and infraspinatus tendon is impinged between the humeral head and glenoid labrum during shoulder abduction and external rotation (late cocking phase in pitching).

3. **Strains and sprain**—if there is a preceding injury or trauma (such as fall, pull, etc.) to the development of shoulder pain, muscle/tendon strains or ligament sprains can be suspected. Rotator cuff strain is one of the most common diagnoses in the shoulder. Deltoid muscle strain is underrecognized but can also cause similar pain as rotator cuff strains. A subdeltoid bursa is located between the rotator cuff tendon and deltoid muscle. As a result, an accompanying bursitis is not uncommon. Acromioclavicular (AC) joint ligament complex sprain is a well-known cause of pain after trauma. Depending on the degree of ligament involvement (coracoclavicular or coracoacromial ligament) and displacement of the clavicle, a grading system (I–VI) exists for AC sprain. Other ligament injuries (glenohumeral [GH] ligaments and coracohumeral ligaments) are underrecognized and not easily detected without advanced imaging. An untreated injury can lead to painful instability later. Other structures commonly injured include the labrum of the glenoid. Depending on the injury pattern, it can cause painful clicking and occasionally mechanical locking. Superior aspect of the labrum (superior labrum anterior and posterior) is a common site for the labral tear, and the presentation can be similar to an AC joint sprain. As degenerative labral pathology is very common, the correlation of the event/injury and the imaging finding is important.

4. **Osteoarthritis**—common locations of osteoarthritis in the shoulder include the AC joint, GH joint, and sternoclavicular (SC) joint. Depending on the location of the joint, the pain can be superior at the AC joint and anteromedial/medial at the SC joint and deep/vague/diffuse in the GH joint osteoarthritis. The pain is gradual in onset, without preceding event or trauma, and worse with activity. Although the disease process is gradual, the patient may feel a relative abrupt onset in the case of flare-up. ROM limitation is more prominent in external rotation than internal rotation (with abduction) as in impingement syndrome. Although ROM restriction varies with the severity of osteoarthritis, it is not as severe as in adhesive capsulitis. Stiffness is present with gradual improvement with movement.

5. **Adhesive capsulitis**—the pain is gradual in onset, poorly localized, initially with overhead activity, or at night, then becomes constant. It is accompanied by painful stiffness then the pain eventually improves gradually. It is more common in females than males, peaks at 40 to 50 years old, and typically presents on the nondominant side. Adhesive capsulitis occurs in up to 20% of patients with diabetes and is more common in patients with thyroid dysfunction, Dupuytren contracture, autoimmune disease, and stroke survivors. Up to 20% to 30% of patients will later develop the symptoms on the unaffected side. Loss of ROM greater than 30 degrees on two planes (frontal, sagittal, or axial) is a commonly used physical examination criterion for diagnosis. Early loss of external rotation is also common. The diagnosis usually requires imaging studies to rule out other mimicking conditions, such as GH osteoarthritis or other inflammatory arthropathies.

6. **Connective tissue disease**—multiple joint arthralgias, fever, weight loss, fatigue, and other systemic symptoms are seen. Rheumatoid arthritis (RA) affects about 1% of adults, with

shoulder joint involvement in 65% to 90% of patients with RA. It increases with advanced disease in the hand/wrist and positive rheumatoid factor. Although effusion is common, it can be subtle and can accompany constitutional symptoms. Extraarticular manifestations such as ocular, pulmonary, and cardiac manifestations are not uncommon.

7. **Polymyalgia rheumatica**—occurs in the older population, average age at diagnosis is over 70 years old, typically presents with subacute or chronic bilateral shoulder pain, significant morning stiffness ($\geq$30 min), and can be aggravated by overhead activity because of subacromial bursitis (frequently coexisting). Bilateral pelvic girdle pain is less common than shoulder pain but occurs in about 50% of patients with polymyalgia rheumatica. It is often self-limiting over months to years. C-reactive protein (CRP) and erythrocyte sedimentation rate (ESR) are significantly elevated.[1]

8. **Idiopathic brachial plexopathy (Parsonage-Turner syndrome)**—rare, but underrecognized disease, with an incidence of 1 to $4/10^5$ per year. It is slightly more common in males than females with a peak incidence between the second and third decades. It presents with severe shoulder pain, frequently 7/10 or higher on a numeric rating scale lasting days or weeks. Typically, the improvement of the pain is followed by weakness and atrophy of the muscle. It is a common cause of scapular winging with involvement of the long thoracic nerve and serratus anterior weakness.[2]

9. **Cervical radiculopathy**—in C5, C6 radiculopathy, the neck pain can radiate down to the shoulder. Typically, the intensity of neck pain is more than or similar to the shoulder pain;however, significant shoulder pain without neck pain is possible. If the pain is reproduced by the cervical spine movement, particularly the Spurling maneuver (cervical extension and lateral flexion), which narrows down the neural foramen, the suspicion for cervical radiculopathy can be higher. It is often difficult to differentiate from cervical facet arthropathy because the referred pain overlaps with radiating pain. The presence of sensory (especially negative symptom/sign) or motor deficits can favor cervical radiculopathy.

10. **Cervical facet arthropathy**—cervical facet arthropathy based on imaging study is prevalent in older adults and increases with age. It is often asymptomatic, and symptomatic arthropathy typically causes pain in the midline neck with/without referred pain. C4–C5 level is the most common level of degenerative changes, and C5–C6 is known to be the most common location of pain with referred pain to upper trapezius and shoulder.[3,4] The pain can be aggravated by cervical spine extension, which is not specific. Reproduction or significant relief of pain with imaging-guided injection is required to confirm facet joint as pain generator.[3,5] Unlike cervical radiculopathy, it lacks focal neurologic deficits.

11. **Myofascial pain syndrome**—arguably the most common cause of the shoulder girdle pain. A patient usually complains of shoulder girdle pain with or without referred pain. Sensory abnormalities, such as tingling paresthesia, can be present. Depending on the involved muscle, pain can be referred to the occiput (trapezius), upper arm, and rarely to the distal upper extremity. The patient does not have a preceding injury or trauma but often complains of increased stress or workload. Headaches may present if suboccipital and trapezius muscles are involved. Referred pain may be felt in upper arms, elbows, and forearms with palpation of the associated trigger points. Physical examination is usually negative other than trigger point palpation with reproduction of symptoms. Skilled palpation techniques may help to identify the areas of trigger points. Abnormal postures and biomechanics are often associated with the development of myofascial pain syndrome, therefore it is important to identify and address it.

12. **Fracture**—history of trauma usually precedes. Examination reveals pain and focal tenderness with limited ROM because of pain. In patients with risk factors, only minor trauma is required to cause fracture. Subtle nondisplaced fractures can be missed without increased suspicion in elderly patients with osteoporosis. Proximal humeral fracture is particularly

common in the elderly after a fall. In contrast, youth throwing athletes can develop an injury at the proximal humeral epiphysis called *little leaguer shoulder*. It can cause disabling pain in the shoulder, especially during throwing motion, and tenderness on the lateral aspect of the proximal humerus is common.

13. **Septic arthritis**—the shoulder is an uncommon location for septic arthritis, 3% to 5% of all septic arthritis, therefore it is underrecognized. It is more common in patients with RA, prosthetic joint, and other risk factors, such as human immunodeficiency virus (HIV). Pain can be exquisite, constant with limited ROM, accompanied by swelling, warmth, and erythema. Because of the lack of typical symptoms and signs initially, delay of diagnosis is common, either by the patient or by healthcare providers. Constitutional symptoms, such as malaise, and low-grade fever may be present. The complete blood count may be normal or show leukocytosis with left shift, but CRP and ESR are frequently elevated.[6]

14. **Charcot neuroarthropathy**[7,8]—rare cause of destructive arthropathy typically related to the syrinx of the spinal cord. Diabetes mellitus is the most common underlying cause of Charcot neuroarthropathy, but more commonly involving the distal lower extremity, such as the foot and ankle. Because of a lack of pain, the patient does not recognize progressive destruction of the humeral head and glenoid until it has progressed significantly. When symptomatic, it presents with shoulder pain with decreased ROM and often with swelling and joint deformity.

15. **Tumor and bony metastasis**—the shoulder region is the third most common site for bone and soft tissue tumors. Primary bony tumors of the shoulder are more likely to be malignant with osteosarcoma and chondrosarcoma, with Ewing sarcoma being the most common.[9] Pain from bony and soft tissue tumors is constant when present, and worse in resting position. Systemic manifestations such as weight loss may accompany.

Case Discussion

Our patient presented with indolent development of symptoms over a few months, suggesting chronicity. An acute traumatic or vascular event is less likely to be the underlying etiology of the patient's presentation. Lack of focal sensory or motor deficit, worsening of pain with shoulder movement (especially overhead activity), and lack of focal neurologic deficit suggests local musculoskeletal pathologies as underlying etiologies.

Recognition of the pain with a specific position can be important information to further localize the lesion. For example, if the pain is reproduced by internal rotation and abduction engaging the supraspinatus or subdeltoid bursa between greater tuberosity and coracoacromial arch, subacromial impingement syndrome should be suspected. If the ROM is limited with pain in multiple directions (planes) of shoulder ROM, capsular or GH joint pathologies, such as adhesive capsulitis or GH arthropathy should be suspected. The characteristics of pain can also be useful information. Persistent pain, even on resting or night pain, may be suggestive of an inflammatory etiology (bursitis and capsulitis)[10] rather than mechanical (tendinopathy by impingement, labral pathology). Lack of symptoms in the contralateral shoulder and other joints are against systemic disease, such as inflammatory arthropathy (RA, polymyalgia rheumatica, etc.). Absence of red flags argues against an infectious underlying etiology or tumors as the underlying cause of pain; however, laboratory tests such as ESR and CRP can be useful if there is any suspicion for an infectious or inflammatory process.

Underlying diabetes mellitus and involvement of the nondominant side with decreased ROM in multiple planes increases the likelihood of adhesive capsulitis as the diagnosis; however, other diagnoses such as GH joint arthropathy or infectious arthropathy should also be ruled out. Other bony or joint pathologies such as avascular necrosis or bony tumor are less likely, and imaging study can be helpful to rule out these conditions.

Objective Data

Complete blood count—within normal limits

Complete metabolic panel—within normal limits

ESR and CRP—within normal limits

X-ray of left shoulder—degenerative changes in the AC joint. Irregularity was noted in the greater tuberosity. The acromion had a hook shape. There was no fracture, dislocation, or osteolytic lesion noted.

Ultrasonography (US) of left shoulder—degenerative changes in the AC joint with capsular bulging. Increased thickness and hypoechogenicity of the supraspinatus tendon with an intact infraspinatus and subscapularis tendon. There was no gross thickening of subacromial bursal tissue or gross effusion in the subacromial bursa or GH joint recess. The long head of the biceps tendon was intact with increased tenosynovial fluid (3 mm). There was increased thickness of the coracohumeral ligament: 4.5 mm, measured on a transverse ultrasound scan of the rotator cuff interval.

Case Discussion

The aforementioned laboratory and imaging data are helpful to further narrow down the differential diagnosis. Because ESR and CRP levels are normal, infectious processes could be eliminated. Primary bony tumors and metastatic lesions are less likely because the patient does not have red flags, and imaging studies did not reveal any lytic or blastic lesions, although early-stage tumors and small soft tissue tumors cannot be completely ruled out.

Clinically, we had a low suspicion for cervical spine–referred pain because the patient did not present with any focal neurological deficits or neck pain. If there is no significant improvement (response) for initial treatment of the local shoulder pathology, additional cervical spine imaging can be useful.

The objective data are notable for x-ray and US findings suggestive of degenerative AC joint disease, rotator cuff tendinopathy (supraspinatus), and adhesive capsulitis (based on the increased thickness of coracohumeral ligament and decreased ROM on multiple planes). It is common to have imaging findings demonstrating multiple musculoskeletal pathologies in any joint–soft tissue complex. Therefore there is increasing emphasis on the correlation between clinical evaluation and radiologic findings. The patient's current clinical findings are more likely secondary to adhesive capsulitis, considering the limited ROM and the nature of pain (constant), rather than secondary to supraspinatus tendinopathy or AC joint pathology. The following is the comprehensive review of shoulder impingement syndrome and adhesive capsulitis.

Review of Proposed Pathology and Pathobiomechanics

Capsule-mediated pain can occur with any directional movement versus pain from impingement syndrome is provoked by the specific movement (internal rotation and abduction in subacromial impingement, external rotation, and abduction in the internal impingement, etc.). The capsulitis develops with/without any clear etiology (secondary and primary/idiopathic), and it usually begins with hypervascular, hypertrophic synovitis with normal capsular tissue. Then the synovitis evolves into pedunculated synovitis, with the development of a perivascular and subsynovial scar. With the synovitis lessening (with hypercellular collagenous tissue), the adhesion becomes mature. This explains the gradual relief of the pain with persistent limitation of ROM.

Primary (idiopathic) adhesive capsulitis can be found more frequently in patients with diabetes (more in type 2 than type 1), as illustrated in this case. Secondary adhesive capsulitis can develop secondary to trauma, surgery, or immobilization.

Although prominent clinical feature can be explained by adhesive capsulitis, underlying rotator cuff tendinopathy cannot be ruled out considering typical US findings, suggestive of supraspinatus tendinopathy.

Subacromial impingement syndrome is the most common impingement syndrome, indicating impingement between the undersurface of the acromion (often extending to coracoacromial ligament/coracoacromial arch) and greater tuberosity. In this case, intermittent pain with overhead activity and supraspinatus tendinopathy can suggest preexisting or concomitant subacromial impingement syndrome. Typical provocation testing (Hawkins Kennedy test with shoulder abduction and internal rotation and Neer arm forward flexion test) is limited because of a painful global decrease in ROM in this patient. Shoulder abduction requires external rotation of the humerus. Previously, thickened coracohumeral and superior GH ligament in the rotator cuff interval (anteriorly located with checking external rotation) was shown to correlate well with the clinical examination finding of decreased ROM among patients with adhesive capsulitis.[11]

Idiopathic adhesive capsulitis is a self-limiting process; however, supraspinatus tendinopathy from subacromial impingement syndrome can be progressive. Therefore it is important to recognize this condition and develop the treatment plan.

Mechanisms for painful impingement were multifactorial, including bony anatomy (hook or flat acromion), GH instability, calcific tendinopathy, fracture in the greater tuberosity with malunion, and mobile os acromiale. Any abnormal biomechanics that decrease the space of impingement during static and dynamic motion can be a culprit, therefore dynamic evaluation during shoulder activity is important to detect abnormal biomechanics. Abnormal biomechanics of scapular position (protracted scapula) or movement (scapular dyskinesia) is associated with impingement syndrome. Tight scapular protractor muscles (pectoralis minor, major) cause anterior tilting of the scapula with an associated decrease in the subacromial space. Scapular dyskinesia secondary to the imbalance between scapular protractor and retractor (rhomboids and middle trapezius muscle) decreases the effective subacromial space during shoulder motion, therefore promoting the impingement.[12,13]

CLINICAL SIGNS AND SYMPTOMS OF ADHESIVE CAPSULITIS AND SHOULDER IMPINGEMENT SYNDROME

Patients with adhesive capsulitis typically present with insidious onset of shoulder pain over several months, often diffusely located, that can be worse at night initially. Pain often interrupts sleep and patients complain of the inability to sleep on the painful side.[14] Pain gradually improves as the stiffness worsens with significant loss of ROM. Although pain is not limited to overhead activity (as in impingement syndrome), it is common to have worsening pain with overhead activity. It is self-limiting, but it takes about 1 to 3 years to resolve the symptom.

Restriction of ROM can be confused with muscle weakness from neurologic disease involving C5–C6, upper trunk brachial plexus, and suprascapular nerve. Passive ROM is usually preserved in the neurologic disorder without pain whereas passive and active ROM are significantly limited in adhesive capsulitis. Sensory deficit other than pain or occasional tingling is not common in musculoskeletal pathologies.[15]

Scapular dyskinesia or paradoxic scapular movement occurs when the patient abducts the arm (exaggerated scapulothoracic movement to compensate the limited GH joint range; opposite to normal 2:1 ratio of GH vs scapulothoracic movement), which can mask the abduction deficit unless undressed.

External rotation of GH joint can be particularly useful considering the thickening of coracohumeral and superior GH ligament in the rotator cuff interval between the supraspinatus and subscapularis in adhesive capsulitis (see Fig. 3.1). Significant difference side to side in the sidearm external rotation test can be useful (Fig. 3.2).

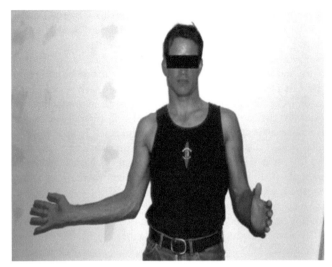

Fig. 3.2 Restriction in external rotation of left glenohumeral joint compared with the right shoulder. (From P.J. McMahon, Adhesive capsulitis, In: Operative Techniques: Shoulder and Elbow Surgery, Elsevier, Philadelphia, 2019, Fig. 39.1.)

Neurologic examination can also be useful to differentiate the other mimicking pathologies, such as brachial plexopathy and C5–C6 radiculopathy. In brachial plexopathy, there is weakness and atrophy beyond the GH joint muscles (such as biceps and forearm muscle and anterior interosseous nerve innervated muscles) although periscapular muscles are the most commonly involved muscles in brachial plexopathy.

C5–C6 radiculopathy can be difficult to rule out and often coexist. If the pain is reproduced by cervical spine range (extension and lateral rotation without GH joint movement) with focal neurologic deficits limited to C5–C6 level, it is reasonable to suspect this diagnosis and confirm it with imaging study and electrodiagnosis.

ULTRASONOGRAPHY

In-office US can be used to evaluate the different underlying pathologies of shoulder pain and is particularly useful for soft tissue pathologies such as rotator cuff tendinopathy, tear, subacromial bursopathy, subcoracoid bursopathy, and some bony pathologies, including AC arthropathy or GH arthropathy, particularly crystal deposition disease.

In adhesive capsulitis, US can confirm the clinical diagnosis of adhesive capsulitis with increased inferior GH ligament, and coracohumeral ligament thickness and the ratio were shown to be correlated with the clinical evaluation.[11] Other typical US findings seen in adhesive capsulitis include effusion in the bicipital tenosynovium because it is the extension of GH joint synovium. Tight space in the joint capsular tenosynovium results in increased effusion in this location.

OTHER IMAGING STUDIES

Plain films are very useful in identifying GH joint bony pathology, fracture, or dislocation, especially if preceding injury or trauma exists.

Routine x-ray includes anteroposterior (internal [for lesser tuberosity lesion and Hill Sach lesion] and external [for greater tuberosity and calcific tendinopathy]) and axillary views (for subluxation and glenoid pathology). If there is trauma preceding the development of the symptom, additional views can be added, such as West Point view (axillary lateral) for Bankart lesion and Striker notch view for Hill Sach lesion. There are additional views available for best visualization of specific structure.

Magnetic resonance imaging (MRI) is the best imaging modality overall for most musculo-skeletal pathologies, and it can be particularly useful in evaluation of intraarticular pathologies, such as labral tear, GH ligament, or intracortical pathologies, such as avascular necrosis or bony or soft tissue tumor.[16] Coronal oblique view is particularly useful in supraspinatus tendon evaluation and axial view for the labral evaluation. Optimal evaluation of labrum and partial rotator cuff tendon tear often requires magnetic resonance arthrogram. In addition, the signal intensity of the periarticular muscle can often provide clues for peripheral nerve disorders (such as brachial plexopathy) or muscle disorders (myotonic dystrophy or facioscapulohumeral dystrophy). Computed tomography (CT) scan is rarely indicated except when MRI is contraindicated or to further evaluate scapular or proximal humeral fracture.

Cervical spine imaging is not necessary as an initial routine workup for shoulder pain unless there is suspicion for cervical spine pathologies. Caution should be taken in interpretation of C-spine images as asymptomatic imaging abnormalities (such as cervical spondylosis, facet arthropathy) are common.

ELECTRODIAGNOSIS

Electrodiagnosis (EMG) test is not necessary to evaluate adhesive capsulitis or shoulder impingement syndrome. It may be indicated if there is any significant sensory or motor deficit, especially weakness or significant atrophy in the periscapular muscle. It is very useful to evaluate brachial plexopathy (idiopathic [Parsonage-Turner syndrome], neurogenic thoracic outlet syndrome, etc.) and cervical radiculopathy involving axonal motor segment. EMG can be limited (normal) in both brachial plexopathy and cervical radiculopathy only involving myelin segment or focal sensory segment.

DISCUSSION

It is important to recognize morbid conditions first. If there is any suspicion for infectious conditions (e.g., septic bursitis), septic GH arthritis, or osteomyelitis with red flags, prompt evaluation and timely management should be done. Other conditions, for example, inflammatory GH arthropathy such as RA, bony tumor or metastatic cancer, and intracortical lesion (avascular necrosis) should benefit from consultation to rheumatology, orthopedic surgery, and oncology for proper management in addition to appropriate pain control and therapy.

Prognosis of idiopathic adhesive capsulitis is generally favorable and self-limiting. It is important to educate the patient about the nature of the conditions and return to unrestricted use of the shoulder as much possible. The goal is to improve the pain and function limited by decreased ROM. These can be achieved mostly by nonoperative management. In this case, it is important to identify and improve scapular dyskinesia and faulty biomechanics to address preexisting shoulder impingement syndrome as well.

INITIAL MANAGEMENT

Maintaining ROM despite the painful limitation should be encouraged (benign neglect). Depending on the severity of the pain, physical therapy can be limited initially. Gentle progressive stretching exercise (e.g., "pendulum exercise," "arm overhead") should be tried after modalities (heating modality) or over-the-counter (OTC) pain medication (Fig. 3.3).

The patient can try OTC transcutaneous electrical stimulation unit for temporary pain relief or can try a heating pad or ice pack depending on the preference. OTC pain patch (lidocaine, salicylate, or capsaicin) can be tried to relieve the pain; however, the efficacy is unknown.

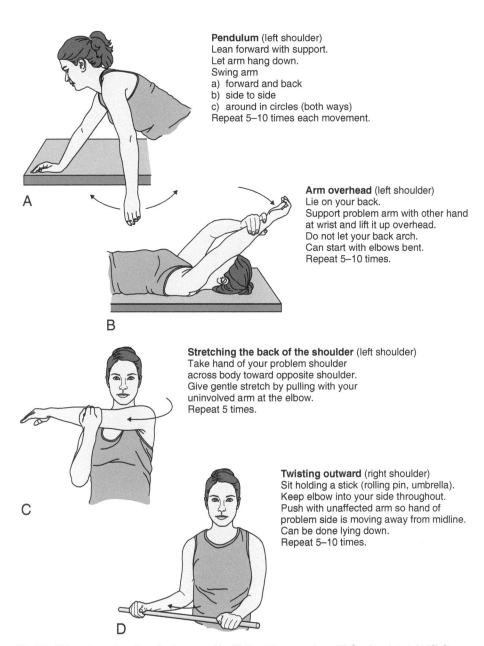

Pendulum (left shoulder)
Lean forward with support.
Let arm hang down.
Swing arm
a) forward and back
b) side to side
c) around in circles (both ways)
Repeat 5–10 times each movement.

Arm overhead (left shoulder)
Lie on your back.
Support problem arm with other hand
at wrist and lift it up overhead.
Do not let your back arch.
Can start with elbows bent.
Repeat 5–10 times.

Stretching the back of the shoulder (left shoulder)
Take hand of your problem shoulder
across body toward opposite shoulder.
Give gentle stretch by pulling with your
uninvolved arm at the elbow.
Repeat 5 times.

Twisting outward (right shoulder)
Sit holding a stick (rolling pin, umbrella).
Keep elbow into your side throughout.
Push with unaffected arm so hand of
problem side is moving away from midline.
Can be done lying down.
Repeat 5–10 times.

Fig. 3.3 Different exercises for adhesive capsulitis. (A) Pendulum exercises. (B) Overhead stretch. (C) Cross-body reach. (D) External rotation.

Continued

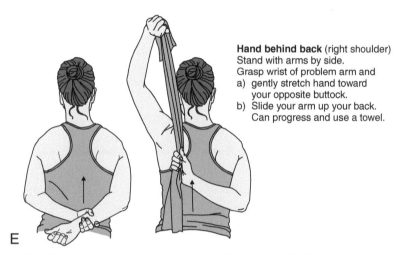

Hand behind back (right shoulder)
Stand with arms by side.
Grasp wrist of problem arm and
a) gently stretch hand toward
   your opposite buttock.
b) Slide your arm up your back.
   Can progress and use a towel.

E

Fig. 3.3, cont'd.   (E) Internal rotation with adduction. (From B.J. Krabak, E.T. Chen, Adhesive capsulitis, In: Essentials of Physical Medicine and Rehabilitation, Elsevier, Philadelphia, 2019, Fig. 11.4.)

Oral Pharmacotherapy

Nonsteroidal antiinflammatory drugs (NSAIDs) can be used as symptomatic relief of pain. Oral steroids with a tapering dose can be used with transient reduction of pain (3–6 weeks) without significant impact on the ROM.[17] Both NSAIDs and oral steroid medications require precautions for elevated cardiovascular risks and gastrointestinal (GI) side effects. Oral steroids are known to affect glucose levels; therefore it is not a great option in this patient with diabetes.

Narcotic analgesics should be reserved for the last resort in the management of adhesive capsulitis considering overall impact on the individual and population health. Given the potential for serious complications, long-term use of NSAIDs and narcotic analgesics should be avoided.

Physical Therapy

A monitored, graduated physical therapy program to restore ROM using manual therapy, scapular stabilization (scapular girdle strengthening and stretching), different modalities (e.g., ultrasound for deep heating modality) for pain relief, and a home exercise program education should be considered. Physical therapy typically focuses on gentle stretching and modality initially, isometric/static exercise, then resistive strengthening exercise (e.g., using resistive band) as ROM improves.[18] Capsular stretch (especially posterior capsular stretching exercise) should be emphasized to increase joint ROM. A Cochrane review reported that a combination of manual therapy and exercise was not as effective as steroid injection in the short term. However, manual therapy and exercise may improve patient-reported outcome and active ROM after the steroid injection.[19]

Injections

Glucocorticosteroids can be injected in the initial painful phase with/without image guidance. Landmark-based injections have varying rates of accuracy depending on the patient's body habitus and experience of the physiatrist. In general, image-guided (either fluoroscopic-guided or ultrasound-guided) steroid injection was more favorable than blind injection for GH joint injection. A retrospective review by Ahn et al. showed early steroid (20 mg of triamcinolone and 8 mL of 1% lidocaine) under US guidance improved short- (1 month) and long-term (12 months) outcome in patients with idiopathic adhesive capsulitis after failed (at least 1 month) conservative treatment.[20] Suprascapular nerve block can be used for pain control as the suprascapular nerve innervated the GH joint capsule.

When the initial injection fails to provide reasonable pain relief, hydrodilation using a larger volume of injectate (up to 50 mL[21] or alternative dose of 20 mL to preserve capsule[22]) can be tried. A mechanical effect to dilate or disrupt (tear) the constricted capsule can be achieved by the injection.

Hyaluronic acid injection can be considered in someone if steroid is contraindicated; however, there is limited supporting evidence in the literature.[23]

Referral to Surgery

If the pain is persistent despite the conservative management, and the quality of life is significantly compromised despite several months of conservative management, referral to surgery can be considered.

Levin et al. reported patients with more severe symptoms initially, younger age at the time of onset, and continuous reduction in ROM despite 4 months of compliant therapy more likely received surgery.[24]

Manipulation under regional or general anesthesia can be used after failed conservative management.

Arthroscopic intervention includes capsular release, capsulotomy, and division, which can provide long-term relief of pain and restoration of ROM. Gallacher et al. compared the arthroscopic capsular release versus hydrodilation and reported significantly higher patient outcome score (the Oxford Shoulder Score) in the surgical group compared with the hydrodilation group, although both groups reported significant improvement.[25]

Summary

This patient presented with insidious onset of chronic shoulder pain, worsening over time, multidirectional restricted ROM with pain, and no focal neurologic deficit outside of the peri-GH joint musculatures. The patient underwent plain x-ray and in-office US, which confirmed the clinical diagnosis of adhesive capsulitis, AC arthropathy, and concomitant supraspinatus tendinopathy. The patient was educated about the favorable nature of the condition and encouraged to maintain the ROM despite the painful limitation. The patient took OTC pain medication (NSAIDs) and was educated on gentle stretching exercises at home. However, because of persistent pain, the patient received an US-guided GH joint steroid injection followed by physical therapy. After the initial US-guided steroid injection, the pain was worsening again after 2 months of significant relief, therefore hydrodilation was tried.

At a follow-up in 3 months, the patient reported persistent relief of pain with significant improvement in her shoulder ROM. The patient does not use NSAIDs or other oral pain medication.

Key Points

- The etiology of the shoulder pain is diverse, and a systematic approach is required.
- A focused history and physical examination can narrow down the differential diagnosis and be helpful in the development of a treatment plan.
- Treatment options should be tailored to individual patients, and conservative managements are often successful.

CLINICAL PEARLS

If the range of motion is limited with pain in multiple directions (planes) of shoulder range of motion, capsular or glenohumeral joint pathologies, such as adhesive capsulitis or glenohumeral arthropathy, should be suspected.

Adhesive capsulitis is self-limiting despite the potentially long duration of symptoms (1–3 years). It is diagnosed clinically by significant loss of range of motion on ≥2 planes (frontal, sagittal, or axial).

Different types of injection (image-guided intracapsular steroid injection, suprascapular nerve block, hydrodilation of the capsule) can be considered in the painful phase, complementary to aggressive capsular stretching exercise.

References

1. C.M. Weyand, J.J. Goronzy, Clinical practice, Giant-cell arteritis and polymyalgia rheumatica, N. Engl. J. Med. 371 (1) (2014) 50–57.
2. N. van Alfen, The neuralgic amyotrophy consultation, J. Neurol. 254 (6) (2007) 695–704.
3. A.C. Gellhorn, J.N. Katz, P. Suri, Osteoarthritis of the spine: the facet joints, Nat. Rev. Rheumatol. 9 (4) (2013) 216–224.
4. A.C. Gellhorn, Cervical facet-mediated pain, Phys. Med. Rehab. Clin. North. Am. 22 (3) (2011) 447–458 viii.
5. G. Cooper, B. Bailey, N. Bogduk, Cervical zygapophysial joint pain maps, Pain Med. 8 (4) (2007) 344–353.
6. I.S. Lossos, O. Yossepowitch, L. Kandel, D. Yardeni, N. Arber, Septic arthritis of the glenohumeral joint, A report of 11 cases and review of the literature, Medicine (Baltim.) 77 (3) (1998) 177–187.
7. N. Hatzis, T.K. Kaar, M.A. Wirth, F. Toro, C.A. Rockwood Jr., Neuropathic arthropathy of the shoulder, J. Bone Joint Surg. Am. 80 (9) (1998) 1314–1319.
8. K.M. Kirksey, W. Bockenek, Neuropathic arthropathy, Am. J. Phys. Med. Rehab. 85 (10) (2006) 862.
9. F.M. Vanhoenacker, K.L. Verstraete, Soft tissue tumors about the shoulder, Semin. Musculoskelet. Radiol. 19 (3) (2015) 284–299.
10. J.S. Lewis, Rotator cuff tendinopathy, Br. J Sport. Med. 43 (4) (2009) 236–241.
11. G.Y. Park, J.H. Park, D.R. Kwon, D.G. Kwon, J. Park, Do the findings of magnetic resonance imaging, arthrography, and ultrasonography reflect clinical impairment in patients with idiopathic adhesive capsulitis of the shoulder? Arch. Phys. Med. Rehab. 98 (10) (2017) 1995–2001.
12. F. Struyf, J. Nijs, J.P. Baeyens, S. Mottram, R. Meeusen, Scapular positioning and movement in unimpaired shoulders, shoulder impingement syndrome, and glenohumeral instability, Scand. J. Med. Sci. Sports 21 (3) (2011) 352–358.
13. A.M. Halder, E. Itoi, K.N. An, Anatomy and biomechanics of the shoulder, Orthop. Clin. North. Am. 31 (2) (2000) 159–176.
14. A.S. Neviaser, R.J. Neviaser, Adhesive capsulitis of the shoulder, J. Am. Acad. Orthop. Surg. 19 (9) (2011) 536–542.
15. H.V. Le, S.J. Lee, A. Nazarian, E.K. Rodriguez, Adhesive capsulitis of the shoulder: review of pathophysiology and current clinical treatments, Shoulder Elbow 9 (2) (2017) 75–84.
16. T.G. Sanders, M.D. Miller, A systematic approach to magnetic resonance imaging interpretation of sports medicine injuries of the shoulder, Am. J Sport. Med. 33 (7) (2005) 1088–1105.
17. R. Buchbinder, S. Green, J.M. Youd, R.V. Johnston, Oral steroids for adhesive capsulitis, Cochrane Database Syst. Rev. 4 (2006) CD006189.
18. H.B.Y. Chan, P.Y. Pua, C.H. How, Physical therapy in the management of frozen shoulder, Singapore Med. J. 58 (12) (2017) 685–689.
19. M.J. Page, S. Green, S. Kramer, et al., Manual therapy and exercise for adhesive capsulitis (frozen shoulder), Cochrane Database Syst. Rev. (8) (2014) CD011275.
20. J.H. Ahn, D.-H. Lee, H. Kang, M.Y. Lee, D.R. Kang, S.-H. Yoon, Early intra-articular corticosteroid injection improves pain and function in adhesive capsulitis of shoulder: 1-year retrospective longitudinal study, Pharm. Manag. PMR 10 (1) (2017) 19–27.

21. J.P. Yoon, S.W. Chung, J.E. Kim, et al., Intra-articular injection, subacromial injection, and hydrodilatation for primary frozen shoulder: a randomized clinical trial, J. Shoulder Elbow Surg. 25 (3) (2016) 376–383.

22. E.S. Koh, S.G. Chung, T.U. Kim, H.C. Kim, Changes in biomechanical properties of glenohumeral joint capsules with adhesive capsulitis by repeated capsule-preserving hydraulic distensions with saline solution and corticosteroid, Pharm. Manag. PMR 4 (12) (2012) 976–984.

23. R. Papalia, A. Tecame, G. Vadala, et al., The use of hyaluronic acid in the treatment of shoulder capsulitis: a systematic review, J. Biol. Regul. Homeostat. Agents. 27 31 (4 Suppl. 2) (2017) 23–32.

24. W.N. Levine, C.P. Kashyap, S.F. Bak, C.S. Ahmad, T.A. Blaine, B. LU, Nonoperative management of idiopathic adhesive capsulitis, J. Shoulder Elbow Surg. 16 (5) (2007) 569–573.

25. S. Gallacher, J.C. Beazley, J. Evans, et al., A randomized controlled trial of arthroscopic capsular release versus hydrodilatation in the treatment of primary frozen shoulder, J. Shoulder Elbow Surg. 27 (8) (2018) 1401–1406

26. S.W. Lee, Musculoskeletal Injuries and Conditions: Assessment and Management, Demos Medical, New York, 2017.

27. B. Goldstein. Shoulder anatomy and biomechanics, Phys. Med. Rehab. Clin. N. Am. 15 (2) (2004) 313–349.

CHAPTER 4

Knee Pain

Dr. Subhadra Nori, MD ▪ Dr. Iris Tian, DO

Case Presentation

A 32-year-old healthy female presents to the Physical Medicine and Rehabilitation (PM&R) clinic with a 2-month history of bilateral knee pain. Denies inciting event or trauma. She does recall picking up running several months ago and runs 1 to 2 miles a day. Pain is dull, aching in nature but at times can be sharp. Pain is localized anteriorly and deep to the patella. Pain is intermittent but worse with negotiating stairs, especially going downstairs, and transitioning from sitting to standing after driving in her car for prolonged periods. Sometimes she notes some effusion in the lateral aspect of her knee at the end of the day. Denies buckling of knees with ambulation or significant effusion. Pain has become slightly worse since onset. She takes Tylenol and Advil occasionally, which provide some relief. She has not tried heat or ice. Pain does not keep her up at night. She has not seen a physician for this pain before coming into your clinic.

  Past medical history: None
  Past surgical history: None
  Allergies: No known drug allergies
  Medications: Tylenol and Advil occasionally
  Social history: Works as an accountant, lives with her boyfriend on third floor of an apartment
     building with elevator access, denies tobacco, alcohol, and illicit drug use

PHYSICAL EXAMINATION

  Vital signs: BP: 132/68 mmHg, RR: 12 breaths/min, PR: 68 per min, T: 97.6°F, Ht: 5'6", Wt: 135
     lbs, BMI: 21.8 kg/m^2
  General: Awake, alert, well-nourished, not in acute distress
  Head, eyes, ears, nose, and throat examination: Extraocular movements intact, moist mucous
     membranes
  Extremities: No edema in bilateral lower extremities
     No atrophy noted in quadriceps or calves

MUSCULOSKELETAL EXAMINATION OF BILATERAL KNEES

  Inspection: No erythema, rashes, surgical scars, bony abnormalities noted in bilateral knees
     No significant genu valgum or varum in knees
  Palpation: No warmth to palpation
  No tenderness to palpation over or surrounding patellar bilaterally
     No tenderness to palpation medial and lateral joint lines, over medial cruciate ligament (MCL)/
        lateral cruciate ligament (LCL) bilaterally
     No tenderness to palpation surrounding quadriceps and patellar tendons (+) Mild tenderness over
        pes anserine in the left knee
  Range of motion (ROM): Full active and passive ROM but pain with 90-degree flexion to maximal
     extension bilaterally
  Provocative: (+) Clarke test bilaterally, (+) mild J-sign noted in the right knee
  Neuro: 5/5 bilateral lower extremities: hip flexion, knee extension/flexion, ankle dorsiflexion/
     plantarflexion, big toe extension
     MSRs 2+ patella, Achilles, no ankle clonus bilaterally
     Sensation intact to light touch bilateral lower extremities
  Gait: Within normal limits, steady, normal cadence
  Tone: Normal throughout bilateral lower extremities
  Labs: None to review

General Discussion

The approach to knee pain is dependent on the location of pain, mechanism of injury (if applicable), and sudden versus insidious onset. Based on the history and exam, it is important to determine whether imaging should be ordered to evaluate for surgical intervention versus more conservative measures. The points to focus on in the physical examination include weightbearing status, ROM testing, provocative maneuvers, and gait mechanics.

DIFFERENTIAL DIAGNOSES

1. Acute injuries
2. Rheumatologic/inflammatory conditions
3. Chronic/overuse injuries

Acute injuries include:

1. **Ligamentous injuries**—anterior cruciate ligament (ACL), posterior cruciate ligament (PCL), MCL, LCL tears. Most common ligamentous injury is to the ACL and is often sports-related with cutting, twisting movements with sudden change in directions. This is often associated with an audible "pop" followed by severe pain, rapid swelling, loss of ROM, and instability with weightbearing. Of note, the "unhappy triad" or O'Donoghue triad involves injury to the ACL, MCL, and medial meniscus.[1,2] The rate of ACL injury for female collegiate athletes is significantly higher, regardless of mechanism of injury, compared with male collegiate athletes in both soccer and basketball.[3,4]
2. **Meniscal injuries**—medial and lateral meniscal tears. Tears usually result from twisting motions at the knee joint and can lead to effusion and tenderness to palpation at the joint line. Most commonly, "locking" occurs particularly at 20 to 45 degrees of extension as the piece of meniscus gets trapped within the joint space. Magnetic resonance imaging (MRI) is helpful and arthroscopy is the standard for diagnosis.[5]
3. **Tendon injuries**—quadriceps or patellar tears or ruptures. Sudden onset of pain with a "pop" that is felt or heard along with swelling and inability to extend the knee. Notable translation of the patella superiorly or inferiorly may be present.
4. **Fractures**—patella, tibial plateau, tibial eminence, tibial tuberosity, femoral condyles. Caused by direct or high impact force that is very painful and patient will have difficulty bearing weight, especially in tibial plateau fractures, and with ROM.[6]
5. **Dislocation**—considered a medical emergency as this can severely compromise blood supplies to the lower extremities. Commonly occurs in motor vehicle collisions where the knee hits the dashboard.

Rheumatologic/inflammatory conditions include:

1. **Rheumatoid arthritis**—autoimmune condition affecting any joint in the body, including the knee which can cause severe pain and swelling.
2. **Infections**—septic arthritis. Symptoms include erythema, rubor, and swollen knee that is very painful. Systemic effects including fevers, chills, and malaise. Diagnosis is through aspiration and fluid analysis.
3. **Gout/pseudogout**—an inflammatory arthritis (high uric acid levels) that commonly occurs in the big toe whereas pseudogout (deposits of calcium pyrophosphate crystals) often occurs in the knees and wrists.

Chronic/overuse injuries include:

1. **Osteoarthritis**—most common form of arthritis that occurs when the protective cartilage that act as shock absorbers deteriorates over time.
2. **Bursitis**—suprapatellar, prepatellar, infrapatellar, pes anserine. Inflammation of the bursa surrounding the patella because of irritation caused by repetitive movements.
3. **Patellar tendonitis**—a chronic condition caused by repetitive flexion motions that is common in cyclist and runners.

4. **Iliotibial band (ITB) syndrome**—runs from the iliac crest to Gerdy tubercle on the tibia and is a key stabilizer for the lateral knee with flexion and extension movements. ITB syndrome is an overuse injury resulting from inflammation and irritation of the ITB as it travels back and forth across the femoral epicondyle.

5. **Patellofemoral pain syndrome (PFPS)**—may be the result of malalignment of the patella caused by muscle imbalances (often weakness of the vastus medialis) or degenerative changes that occur on the posterior articular cartilage of the patella over time from overuse (chrondromalacia patellae).[19]

Other Considerations:

1. Biomechanics play a huge role in knee pain and any subtle change in movement, such as leg-length discrepancies or change in gait, may induce new onset knee pain.

2. Excess weight and obesity can contribute to knee pain over time and increase the risk of knee osteoarthritis.

When examining the knee, it may also be helpful to focus on the location of pain to narrow down your differential diagnoses. Refer to Table 4.1, "Overview of Common Structures in Knee Pain and Provocative Tests."

1. Anterior
2. Posterior
3. Medial
4. Lateral

Case Discussion

Because the patient presents without trauma and an insidious onset of pain, we are less concerned about a severe injury requiring immediate or urgent surgical intervention, but they should be ruled out based on history, physical examination, and prudent clinical judgment. One of the most important parts of the examination includes having the patient walk and analyzing the gait with attention to genu varum/valgum and degree of pronation/supination of the foot. Pain appears to correlate with an increase in activity level as she started running and worse with transitional movements from prolonged flexion to extension.

When evaluating the knee joint, consider how the joint above and below may affect gait mechanics. Sometimes pain in the knees can be referred from the hip. Pes planus or pes cavus may also play a role as excessive pronation leads to compensatory internal rotation of the tibia and femur and excessive supination places more stress on the patellofemoral joint.

Objective data

There is no laboratory work to review, but if there is concern for inflammation or infections, erythrocyte sedimentation rate (ESR) and C-reactive protein (CRP) should be obtained along with other labs including rheumatologic panel, uric acid levels, etc. as indicated.

X-ray of knees—rule out degenerative changes and fractures in acute knee injuries based on the Ottawa knee rules:

- >55 years of age, tenderness at the fibular head, isolated tenderness of patella, inability to flex knee >90 degrees, inability to bear weight × 4 steps[7]

MRI of knees—rule out ligamentous and meniscal injuries given relevant history and physical exam.

The aforementioned laboratory and imaging data are helpful to further narrow down the differential diagnosis. There are no gross deformities so dislocation of the knee is ruled out. There is no effusion or warmth to palpation noted so septic joint and gout/pseudogout are not likely. Because the patient is able to weight bear without pain and denies buckling of her knees with ambulation, fractures, complete ruptures of the quadriceps or patellar tendons, and ligamentous tears (ACL, PCL, LCL, MCL) are less likely. Given her age, osteoarthritis is also unlikely. Patient recently started running, which points to the differential diagnoses that are likely caused by chronic/overuse injuries including tendonitis and patellofemoral syndrome.

TABLE 4.1 ■ **Overview of Common Structures in Knee Pain and Provocative Tests**

Structure	Mechanism of Injury	Location of Pain	Provocative Test
Anterior cruciate ligament (ACL)	- Twisting, cutting motions (sudden change in direction where lower leg is fixed) often sports-related - 70% of cases noncontact[21]	- Deep within knee, severe	Lachman Anterior drawer Pivot shift
Posterior cruciate ligament (PCL)	- Direct impact to the anterior aspect of the proximal tibia with knee in flexed position and ankle plantarflexed - Often in dashboard injuries in motor vehicle collisions - Often occurs with other ligamentous injuries[20]	- Deep within knee (usually minimal/ subtle symptoms in isolated injuries)	Posterior drawer Posterior Lachman Posterior sag sign Dial/tibial external rotation
Medial cruciate ligament (MCL)	- Noncontact hyperextension or varus stress - Often occurs with ACL and medial meniscal injuries as part of "unhappy triad"	- Medial to medial joint line	Valgus stress Swain Anteromedial drawer
Lateral cruciate ligament (LCL)	- Direct impact to the anteromedial knee and posterolateral corner - Noncontact hyperextension or varus stress	- Lateral to lateral joint line	Varus stress Anterolateral drawer
Meniscus	- Twisting motion with varus/ valgus forces	- Over medial or lateral joint lines	McMurray Apley compression Thessaly Bounce home Childress/"duck" walk
Patellofemoral joint	- Overuse, commonly lateral tracking of patella caused by muscle imbalances	- Anterior knee pain with excess weight or stress on the patellofemoral joint (squatting, running, kneeling)	Squatting Clarke J sign Patellar tilt

Data from [2, 9, 10, 12, 19]

Review of Proposed Pathology and Pathobiomechanics

PFPS is the most common cause of anterior knee pain. Many structures are involved in tracking of the patellofemoral joint, including the patellar and quadriceps tendons, medial and lateral retinaculum, ITB, and vastus medialis and lateralis muscles. Any change in gait mechanics can create imbalances leading to abnormal tracking over the femoral condyles, which leads to pain over time. A common cause is lateral tracking of the patella caused by the vastus lateralis overpowering the vastus medialis oblique (VMO) and excessive loading onto the knee joint with running and squatting. A hypertonic ITB or lateral retinaculum may also cause lateral tracking of the patella. A wider Q angle was once thought to be a major risk factor for PFPS; however, recent reviews show it is not a significant factor.[8] Other risk factors include knee hyperextension, lateral tibial torsion, genu valgum or varus, or hypertonic hamstrings or gastrocnemius muscles.

Clinical Signs and Symptoms of Patellofemoral Pain Syndrome

Patients commonly present with anterior knee pain that is worse with activities, which increase compressive forces onto the patellofemoral joint, such as squatting, stairs, running, kneeling, and prolonged sitting.

Main Provocative Tests on Physical Examination

There are many provocative maneuvers for PFPS. Based on a systematic review with metaanalysis of the clinical diagnostic tests for PFPS, the squatting test and patellar tilt tests had values that show a trend, but not clear evidence, for the diagnosis of PFPS.[9]

Squatting—anterior pain with active squatting presents the highest sensitivity as this significantly increases the load on the knee joint, exacerbating symptoms.[10]

Clarke—start with patient supine with knee in full extension and relaxed. Place index finger and thumb over superior border of the patella and ask patient to contract quadriceps (or bring knee to the table). Pain indicates positive test.

J sign—lateral patellar tracking during the terminal phase of extension with active flexion to full extension of the knee by the patient.

Patellar tilt—with the patient's knee extended, grasp patella between thumb and forefinger. The medial aspect of the patella is compressed posteriorly causing the lateral aspect to elevate. If lateral aspect does not elevate, this is an indication of tightness of the lateral structures/retinaculum of the patella.

Imaging Studies

Plain films are not usually helpful but may rule out degenerative changes, including osteoarthritis, and in some cases may show chondromalacia over time.

MRI is useful to rule out cartilages or ligamentous causes of knee pain.

Imaging is not typically needed for diagnosis but should be considered if there was direct trauma to the knee or if significant effusion is seen on examination. It may also be considered if the patient is over 50 years of age or if patient does not improve with conservative management in 8 to 12 weeks.[11]

Grading of Meniscal Injuries[12,13]:

Grade 1: Few fibers are injured with local tenderness, no instability

Grade 2: More extensive fiber damage and tenderness, no instability or mild instability, abnormal motion

Grade 3: Complete tear with notable instability, commonly associated with ligamentous injury especially ACL tears[12]

- Instability grades based on severity with valgus stress examination in 30-degree knee flexion:
  - 1+ with 3–5 mm, 2+ with 6–10 mm, 3+ with >10 mm medial joint space opening

Discussion

PFPS is a common result of overuse injuries especially with running and squatting. Because of the many factors that contribute to PFPS, a multifaceted exercise program is important. Most patients improve with rest from strenuous training and a therapy program focused on proximal muscle strengthening (quadriceps).

Conservative Treatment

Rest: From strenuous training, such as running/jogging, to relieve stress on the patellofemoral joint.

Physical therapy: The most effective and strongly supported treatment for PFPS is a 6-week physiotherapy program focusing on strengthening the quadriceps and hip muscles and stretching the quadriceps, ITB, hamstrings, and hip flexors.[14] Isometric exercises are helpful in the beginning by decreasing the stress on the patellofemoral joint as the knees are fully extended leading to pain-free strengthening exercises. Although it is difficult to isolate the VMO, it may be effective to exercise at 0 to 30 degrees of flexion.[15]

Manual therapy may help relax hypertonic muscles, including hamstrings, quadriceps, and ITBs. Although patellar taping and bracing have shown some benefits, the data are inconclusive.[14] Both may still be helpful to reduce lateral patellar tracking and decrease pain. If there is mild effusion, ice may help. It may also be helpful for the therapist to correct the patient's form when squatting, such as making sure the knee does not go past the toes as this places higher mechanical forces on the patellofemoral joint.

Orthotics: May be considered if there is a leg-length discrepancy but it must be noted that most people have naturally compensated for this so adding orthotics may lead to worsening pain by changing the gait mechanics.

Acupuncture: There is evidence in reducing pain in patients with knee osteoarthritis.

Supplements: Glucosamine and chondroitin supplements for arthritis, vitamin D for proximal muscle strengthening, and vitamin C for connective tissue health have inconclusive evidence.

Weight loss: Reduces the overall weight placed on the knees with ambulation as excess weight alternates gait mechanics and places more stress on the knees leading to worsening knee pain. A recent metaanalysis demonstrated that knee osteoarthritis risk increased almost exponentially according with the increase of BMI.[16] For each pound of weight lost, there is a fourfold reduction in the load exerted on the knee per step during daily activities.[17]

PHARMACOTHERAPY

Nonsteroidal antiinflammatory drugs (NSAIDs): There is limited information regarding use of NSAIDs but may be considered for short-term management while patient undergoes physical therapy.[18]

Interventions

Injections: These are not recommended for PFPS; however, corticosteroids and lubricants, such as hyaluronate gel may be considered for mild to moderate osteoarthritis that do not improve with therapy and other modalities.

Aspiration: This can be diagnostic and therapeutic for patients with significant effusion and to rule out septic joint or gout/pseudogout.

Arthroscopy: This is a common, minimally-invasive surgical procedure that is diagnostic, as well as therapeutic (small pieces of bone or cartilage may be removed).

Ligamentous reconstruction: ACL reconstruction is the most commonly reconstructed ligament with grafts taken from the quadriceps, hamstring, or patellar tendons.

Partial/total knee replacements: Reserved for severe osteoarthritis affecting ambulation, quality of life, and activities of daily living.

Summary

We presented a case of a 32-year-old woman with bilateral knee pain. PFPS is the most common cause of anterior knee pain. The patellar and quadriceps tendons, medial and lateral retinaculum, iliotibial band, and vastus medialis and lateralis muscles are responsible for patellar tracking. Any imbalances in the gait mechanics can lead to abnormal tracking of the patella over the femoral condyles, which leads to pain over time. A lateral tracking of the patella caused by the vastus lateralis overpowering the VMO and excessive loading onto the knee joint with running and squatting is more common. Treatment includes NSAIDS, taping, and injections with steroids.

Key Points

- Patients with knee pain should be carefully assessed because the etiology can be diverse and complex.
- Careful attention should be placed to all elements of the history and examination.
- Treatment options should be tailored to individual patients and special consideration given to the activity level of the individual and whether return to work or sports is involved.

References

1. O.E. Olsen, G. Myklebust, L. Engebretsen, et al., Injury mechanisms for anterior cruciate ligament injuries in team handball: a systematic video analysis, Am. J. Sport Med 32 (4) (2004) 1002–1012.
2. K.D. Shelbourne, P.A. Nitz, The O'Donoghue triad revisited Combined knee injuries involving anterior cruciate and medial collateral ligament tears, Am. J. Sport Med. 19 (5) (1991) 474–477.
3. J. Agel, E. Arendt, B. Bershadsky, Anterior cruciate ligament injury in national collegiate athletic association basketball and soccer: a 13 year review, Am. J. Sports. Med. 33 (4) (2005) 524–530.
4. L.Y. Griffin, J. Kercher, N. Rossi, Risk and gender factors for noncontact anterior cruciate ligament injury, In: C.C. Prodromos, S.M. Howell, F.H. Fu, et al., (Eds.), Anterior Cruciate Ligament, Saunders, Philadelphia, 2018.
5. V.S. Nikolaou, E. Chronopoulos, C. Savvidou, et al., MRI efficacy in diagnosing internal lesions of the knee: a retrospective analysis, J. Trauma Manag. Outcomes 2 (2008) 4.
6. D.A. Wiss, J.T. Watson, E.E. Johnson, Fractures of the knee. Fractures in Adults, 4e, Lippincott-Raven, Philadelphia, 1996.
7. I.G. Stiell, G.A. Wells, R.H. Hoag, et al., Implementation of the Ottawa Knee Rule for the use of radiography in acute knee injuries, J. Am. Med. Assoc. 278 (1997) 2075–2079.
8. L.A. Bolgla, M.C. Boling, An update for the conservative management of patellofemoral pain syndrome: a systematic review of the literature from 2000 to 2010, Int. J. Sports Phys. Ther. 6 (2011) 112–125.
9. G.S. Nunes, E.L. Stapait, M.H. Kirsten, et al., Clinical test for diagnosis of patellofemoral pain syndrome: systematic review with meta-analysis, Phys. Ther. Sport. 14 (2013) 54–59.
10. C. Cook, E. Hegedus, R. Hawkins, F. Scovell, D. Wyland, Diagnostic accuracy and association to disability of clinical test finding associated with patellofemoral pain syndrome, Physiother. Can. 62 (2010) 17–24.
11. S. Dixit, J.P. DiFiori, M. Burton, et al., Management of patellofemoral pain syndrome, Am. Fam. Physician 75 (2007) 194–202.
12. J.C. Hughston, J.R. Andrews, M.J. Cross, A. Moschi, Classification of knee ligament instabilities. Part I. The medial compartment and cruciate ligaments, J. Bone Joint Surg. Am. 58 (2) (1976) 159–172.
13. H. Makhmalbaf, O. Shahpari, Medial collateral ligament injury; a new classification based on mri and clinical findings, A guide for patient selection and early surgical intervention, Arch. Bone Jt. Surg. 6 (1) (2018) 3–7.
14. J.A. Rixe, J.E. Glick, J. Brady, et al., A review of the management of patellofemoral pain syndrome, Phys. Sportsmed 41 (2013) 19–28.

15. Bolgla L, Malone T. Research review: exercise prescription and patellofemoral pain: evidence for rehabilitation, J. Sport. Rehabil. 14 (1) (2005) 72–88.

16. Z.-Y. Zhou, Y.K. Liu, H.L. Chen, F. Liu, Body mass index and knee osteoarthritis risk: a dose-response meta-analysis, Obesity 22 (10) (2014) 2180–2185.

17. S.P. Messier, D.J. Gutekunst, C. Davis, P. DeVita, Weight loss reduces knee-joint loads in overweight and obese older adults with knee osteoarthritis, Arthritis Rheum. 52 (7) (2005) 2026–2032.

18. H.J. McGowan, A. Beutler, Patellofemoral syndrome. Essential Evidence Plus Web site. Available at: http://www.essentialevidenceplus.com. (Accessed 8 August 2019).

19. C. Cook, L. Mabry, M.P. Reiman, E.J. Hegedus, Best tests/clinical findings for screening of patellofemoral pain syndrome: A systematic review, Physiotherapy 98 (2012) 93–100.

20. M.S. Schulz, K. Russe, A. Weiler, H.J. Eichhorn, M.J. Strobel, Epidemiology of posterior cruciate ligament injuries, Arch. Orthopaed. Trauma Surg. 123 (4) (2003) 186–191.

21. C.C. Teitz, Video analysis of ACL injuries, In: L.Y. Griffin (Ed.), Prevention of Noncontact ACL Injuries, American Academy Orthopaedic Surgeons, Rosemont, IL, 2001.

CHAPTER 5

Hand and Wrist Pain

Dr. Se Won Lee, MD ▪ Dr. Reina Nakamura, DO

Case Presentation

A 54-year-old, right-hand dominant female presents to the Physical Medicine and Rehabilitation (PM&R) clinic with right hand and wrist pain. She describes her pain as aching. The pain began gradually about 9 months ago without preceding injury or trauma. She indicates the pain is deep in the wrist and worse in the radial aspect. The pain is aggravated by using her right hand at work. She takes an occasional ibuprofen, which seems to help temporarily.

There is intermittent tingling in the right hand and fingers; however, she is unable to specify location of paresthesia (diffuse as per patient). She denies any significant neck, shoulder, or elbow pain. She was seen by her primary care doctor who referred her to the clinic.

Past medical history: She has history of increased cholesterol for 5 years. She had menopause 1 year ago.

Social history: She works as an executive secretary, and lives with family in a house with 12 steps. She has a 23-year-old son and 21-year-old daughter.

Past surgical history: None

Allergies: No known drug allergy

Medications: Lovastatin 40 mg daily and ibuprofen 400 mg as needed

BP: 128/76 mmHg, RR: 16/min, PR: 62 per min, Temp: 97° F, Ht: 5'5", Wt: 160 lbs, BMI: 26.6 kg/m^2

General: Well built, well nourished, in no acute distress. She is alert, oriented to person, place, and time

Extremities: No edema, skin rashes/erythema, or surgical scars. No gross deformity of upper and lower extremities.

HEENT: Normal extraocular movements, symmetric face, no ptosis, tongue midline.

NEUROMUSCULOSKELETAL EXAMINATION

Inspection: No gross muscle atrophy other than equivocal thenar eminence flattening. Equivocal shoulder sign (at first carpometacarpal joint) suggestive of first metacarpal dorsoradial subluxation.

Range of motion (ROM): Neck, shoulder, elbow are within functional limits. Full range of wrist with mild discomfort at end range of extension and radial deviation.

Motor examination: 5−/5 right thumb abduction with pain. All other muscles (in both upper and lower extremities): 5/5 strength.

Deep tendon reflexes: 2+ in biceps, triceps, and brachioradialis bilaterally. Negative Hoffman test bilaterally.

Sensory examination: Intact to light touch and pinprick in all dermatomes of bilateral upper extremities.

Tone: Normal

Gait: Within normal limits

Provocation tests for hand and wrist

Finkelstein test: Negative

First carpometacarpal joint grind test: Pain in the joint

Watson test (scaphoid shift test): Negative

Lichtman test for midcarpal instability: Negative

Lunate-triquetral ballottement test (Reagan test): Negative

Piano key sign for radioulnar joint instability: Negative

Ulnar styloid triquetral impaction test: Negative

Labs: White blood cell (WBC): 6800 cell/mL, hemoglobin (Hg):12.0 g/dL

General Discussion: General Approach to Wrist and Hand Pain

Initial approach should focus on differentiating musculoskeletal from neuropathic pain generators. Typically, pain description, such as pins/needle, burning, "shooting," and/or numbness indicate neuropathic pain in origin. In contrast, pain characterized as aching, deep, or sore is more representative of musculoskeletal pain. However, chronic musculoskeletal pathology can have mixed features. Musculoskeletal pathology can be further classified by location of pain and point of maximal tenderness (Table 5.1). Etiologies of neuropathic pain can be further classified by the pattern of symptom distribution; diffuse (peripheral polyneuropathy) versus localized (mononeuropathy [entrapment neuropathy]) versus regional (cervical radiculopathy or brachial plexopathy). Less commonly, referred pain from proximal musculoskeletal pathology can mimic neuropathic pain generators.

Gradual onset of chronic wrist and hand pain indicates degenerative or repetitive overuse injury as the underlying mechanism for pain. In contrast, traumatic, vascular, or acute inflammatory processes occur abruptly with immediate or rapid onset. Although serious life-threatening pathologies are less common in the wrist and hand, it is important to recognize red flags, such as history of trauma/puncture and increased external compression, requiring urgent workup and treatment.[1]

Focused physical examination of hand and wrist starts with inspection. Presence of skin lesions (erythema or rash) provides valuable information indicating inflammatory/rheumatologic, vascular, or infectious etiologies. Gross deformity of the hand and wrist suggests underlying chronic destructive pathology or muscle agonist/antagonist imbalance. Common deformities from rheumatoid arthritis (RA) include ulnar deviation of fingers and wrist, joint swelling (Bouchard node in proximal interphalangeal joint and Heberden nodes in distal interphalangeal joint), and finger deformity (Boutonniere or Swan neck deformity). Wartenberg sign (little finger abduction), ulnar claw hand, or benediction sign can be easily recognized in patients with ulnar neuropathy. In addition, it is important to evaluate proximal segments of upper extremities such as elbow, shoulder, and neck.

Significant atrophy of thenar, hypothenar, and/or intrinsic muscles indicates underlying neurologic etiologies. Lower motor neuron disease is favored over upper motor neuron disease, although mild disuse atrophy can occur in chronic painful musculoskeletal conditions. Pattern of atrophy can help the clinician develop and narrow down differential diagnoses.

Mild swelling of the hand and wrist can be easily missed, similar to mild atrophy of the hand and wrist muscles. Swelling may be present in multiple structures (joint, tendon/tenosynovium, or subcutaneous/vascular).

Passive and active ROM of the wrist, hand, and fingers should be examined. ROM of the thumb is particularly complicated, including flexion/extension, abduction/adduction, and opposition/reposition (Fig. 5.1). Flexion/extension occurs in parallel to the palmar plane, abduction/adduction is perpendicular or orthogonal to the palmar plan, and opposition is the combined movement of flexion and abduction.

Systematic palpation provides important clues for local pain generators. Several bony landmarks are useful to remember. At the level of the distal wrist crease, distal pole of the scaphoid and pisiform are easily palpated. The scaphoid is located radially, and the pisiform ulnarly (Fig. 5.2). At the proximal border of the first metacarpal bone, the trapezio-first metacarpal joint (often recognized as ridge of the shoulder sign) is palpable. Rotation of the tip of the thumb can be useful to identify the trapezio-first metacarpal joint with differential rotation (more rotation in the first metacarpal bone vs less mobile trapezium). Distal crease also overlaps with proximal entrance of carpal tunnel. In carpal compression test and Tinel sign, the compression site should be immediately distal to the distal wrist crease.

The pattern and the degree of weakness of muscle strength are useful for differential diagnosis. Weakness secondary to musculoskeletal pain is usually mild from extended disuse, and located around the painful structure rather than following peripheral nerve or myotomal patterns. Except

TABLE 5.1 ▦ **Differential Diagnosis Based on the Location of Pathology**

Region	Structure	Pathologies
Dorsoradial	Bone	First carpometacarpal (CMC) osteoarthritis (OA): MC site for hand OA First metacarpophalangeal, wrist (radial-scaphoid) and scaphoid-trapezium OA Scaphoid fracture, nonunion
	Tendons	de Quervain tenosynovitis involving first dorsal extensor compartment Intersection syndrome; 4–8 cm proximal to radial styloid Extensor digitorum brevis manus syndrome (accessory muscle)
	Nerve	Superficial radial neuropathy
Middorsal	Bone, joint structures	Ganglion; most common (MC) from scapholunate joint Scapholunate ligament sprain, dissociation/instability Carpal boss
	Tendon	Extensor pollicis longus, extensor indicis, or extensor digitorum tendinopathy, tenosynovitis, tear Distal intersection syndrome (between third dorsal extensor compartment and second dorsal extensor compartment intersection distal to the Lister tubercle)
Dorsoulnar	Bone	Arthropathy involving radioulnar joint and CMC joint (triquetrum, hamate, fourth and fifth metacarpal bone) Ulnar triquetral impingement Triangular fibrous cartilage complex (TFCC) lesion
	Tendons	Extensor carpi ulnaris tendinopathy, stenosing tenosynovitis, subluxation/dislocation, tear
Volar radial	Bone	OA of first CMC joint. Wrist and MCP arthropathy Scaphoid cyst/fracture
	Tendons	de Quervain tenosynovitis Flexor carpi radialis tendinopathy Ganglion cyst originated from flexor tendon Linburg-Comstock syndrome (anomalous tendon slip from the flexor pollicis longus to flexor digitorum profundus [to second digit]) Trigger finger (stenosing tenosynovitis) at the A1 pulley
Midvolar	Bone	Arthropathy involving radiocarpal, carpal and second to fourth MCP joints
	Carpal tunnel	Carpal tunnel syndrome (often diffuse)
	Tendon	Trigger finger Linburg-Comstock syndrome
Volar ulnar	Bone	Radioulnar arthropathy/instability, TFCC lesion Pisotriquetral arthritis, ulnotriquetral impingement syndrome, fourth or fifth MCP arthropathy, hook of hamate fracture, fracture of metacarpal bone
	Tendons	Flexor carpi ulnaris tendinopathy Trigger finger
	Nerve	Ulnar neuropathy

Data from [23], [24], [25], [26]

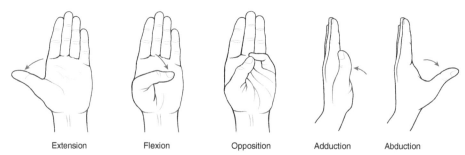

Extension   Flexion   Opposition   Adduction   Abduction

Fig. 5.1 Movements of the thumb. (From T. Klonisch, S. Hombach-Klonisch, J. Peeler, Sobotta Clinical Atlas of Human Anatomy, 1 volume, Elsevier, Munich, Germany, 2019.)

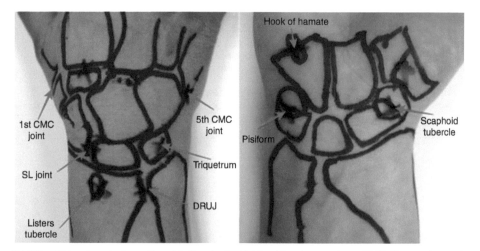

Fig. 5.2 Wrist surface anatomy. Dorsal (*left*) and volar (*right*) wrist surface anatomy. *CMC,* Carpometacarpal; *DRUJ,* distal radioulnar joint; *SL,* scapholunate. (From A.W. Newton, D.H. Hawkes, V. Bhalaik. Clinical examination of the wrist. Orthop. Trauma. 31 (4) (2017) 237–247.)

for muscles in the thenar eminence, most intrinsic hand muscles are innervated by the ulnar nerve. Ulnar nerve lesion can be suspected if there is intrinsic muscle weakness, especially of power grip, such as hook and cylindric grip.

For sensory examination, understanding the difference between peripheral nerve lesions and root lesions can be useful in arriving at the differential diagnosis. Splitting of sensation in the fourth digit in peripheral nerve lesions (either median or ulnar nerve lesion) versus no splitting in C8 radiculopathy is helpful information. However, normal variation of sensory nerve distribution should be acknowledged. Examination of light touch, vibration, two-point discrimination rather than pinprick, and temperature sensation may provide more information in entrapment neuropathy, which typically involves large fibers. Bilateral symptoms with upper motor neuron complaints, such as unsteadiness or gait dysfunction, Hoffman sign, or plantar scratch reflex (Babinski sign), can be useful.

Common Differential Diagnoses for Wrist and Hand Pain

1. **Entrapment neuropathy**—carpal tunnel syndrome is the most common entrapment neuropathy, with a prevalence of about 3%. Patients present with positive sensory (tingling,

paresthesia, pins/needle sensation, and/or pain) or negative sensory (numbness) symptoms in the distribution of median nerve distal to the carpal tunnel. Thenar eminence is spared because the palmar cutaneous branch courses superficial (outside) to the carpal tunnel. Symptoms are typically located in radial 3.5 fingers, with sparing of ulnar side of fourth digit. Because anatomic variation of digital nerve distribution exists, the presentation can vary.

Typically, symptoms are gradual or insidious in onset. However, with additional minor injury or trauma, some patients may report relatively abrupt onset. Symptoms are worse at night and can interfere with sleep by waking the patient. Shaking hands when symptoms occur, known as *Flicker sign*, often improves symptoms.

Ulnar neuropathy at the wrist (Guyon canal) is not as common as ulnar neuropathy at the elbow. Ulnar neuropathy at the wrist presents with sensory and/or motor deficits depending on the location of the lesion in Guyon canal. Because sensory symptoms are underrecognized, presentation is often delayed until significant atrophy of intrinsic hand muscles occurs.

2. **Tendinopathy or tenosynovitis**—pain from tendons and tenosynovial pathology is common in the hand and wrist, typically associated with overuse or repetitive injury. Focal, reproducible pain with exertion (resisted muscle contraction) or stretching is the hallmark physical examination finding of tendinopathy or tenosynovitis. Focal swelling of the tendon or tenosynovium may be present. The most common tendinopathy in the wrist is de Quervain disease, tendinopathy/tenosynovitis of first dorsal extensor compartment (abductor pollicis longus and extensor pollicis brevis). There is pain in the radial aspect of the wrist, in the vicinity of radial styloid process. Tendinopathy/tenosynovitis of extensor carpi ulnaris and flexor carpi ulnaris (FCU) can be suspected in the dorsal-ulnar and volar-ulnar aspect of the wrist.

3. **Strains, sprains, and tear**—localized wrist and hand pain is common following an injury of muscle/tendon (strain) or ligament (sprain). Tenderness of the injured structure can be appreciated with or without ecchymosis and/or swelling depending on the degree of injury. Typically, there are no neurologic symptoms. Ligament sprains include gamekeeper thumb, involving ulnar collateral ligament of first metacarpophalangeal joint or jammed finger involving collateral ligament in the proximal interphalangeal joint. Ligament sprain of carpal bones such as scapholunate, lunate-triquetrum ligament is often underrecognized, later developing into chronic pain and instability.

4. **Osteoarthritis**—most common location of osteoarthritis (OA) in the upper extremity is the hand, particularly in the first carpometacarpal (CMC) joint (trapezio-first metacarpal joint). The radiographic evidence of arthritis is common in middle-aged or elderly (up to 36%), and is more common in females than in males.[2] Symptoms can be vague and confused with other commonly coexisting pain generators that present similarly, such as carpal tunnel syndrome and de Quervain disease. Pain from OA is typically intermittent during early stage of disease, becoming more constant in advanced stages. Pain is aggravated by functional activities requiring axial loading of the joint, especially smaller grip. Subtle swelling of the joint may be present, with radial-dorsal subluxation of the first metacarpal bone (shoulder sign). Stiffness accompanies pain, although not as prolonged as with RA. ROM with axial loading (CMC grind test) reproduces the pain.

5. **Rheumatoid arthritis**—affects an estimated 1% of adults. The disease is two to three times more common in females, with peak onset between 35 and 60 years.[3] RA frequently involves multiple small joints, particularly metacarpophalangeal joints, and proximal interphalangeal joints, typically in both hands.[4] The onset of pain is gradual, typically over weeks to months. Prolonged stiffness lasting greater than 1 hour is common. Swelling of the joint (synovitis) and tenosynovium (tenosynovitis) cause focal, multifocal, or regional swelling. In the early stages, swelling can be difficult to identify without imaging modalities, such as ultrasonography and magnetic resonance imaging (MRI). Initially, symptoms may improve with activity. Because

carpal tunnel syndrome frequently coexists, owing to hyperplastic synovium and thickened transcarpal ligament, the patient may also have sensory symptoms. With prolonged inflammation of tendon/tenosynovium in RA, tear or rupture of tendons is not unusual, which can be mistaken as focal motor deficit from neurologic disorders.

6. **Chondrocalcinosis**[26,27]—the wrist is the second most common location for calcium pyrophosphate dihydrate deposition (CPPD) following the knee joint. Pseudogout is the most common form of crystal deposition disease in the wrist, often involving both wrists and hands. The onset begins between 40 and 50 years of age, typically affects elderly, and is more common in females than males. Other crystal deposition diseases such as gout and hydroxyapatite crystal deposition disease are rare in the wrist. The most common location for CPPD is triangular fibrous cartilaginous complex (TFCC), followed by scaphoid-trapezial-trapezoidal joint. It is associated with other arthropathies, such as OA, RA, and hyperparathyroidism. Typical presentation is with acute pain with swelling, but some are asymptomatic. Minor trauma may act as a trigger of symptoms. In two-thirds of patients, the condition is bilateral.

7. **Psoriatic arthropathy**—an underrecognized inflammatory arthropathy that presents with pain, deformity, redness, and swelling of the fingers (dactylitis). Deformity of fingers is not uncommon, including dactylitis and arthritis mutilans (marked bone resorption or osteolysis with telescoping digits).[5,6] Psoriatic arthropathy often accompanies spondyloarthropathy with low back pain and enthesopathy, such as insertional Achilles tendinopathy or plantar fasciitis.

8. **Bursitis**—uncommon in the wrist and hand, adventitial (acquired, not from native bursa) bursal inflammation should be included in the differential diagnosis for pain with or without focal swelling. Intersection syndrome between first dorsal extensor compartment (abductor pollicis long [APL] and extensor pollicis brevis [EPB]) and second dorsal extensor compartment (extensor carpi radialis longus [ECRL] and brevis [ECRB]) is located approximately 7 to 10 cm proximal to the radial styloid process. Less well known is distal intersection syndrome between second dorsal extensor compartment and third dorsal extensor compartment (extensor pollicis longus) found distal to Lister tubercle on the dorsum of the hand. Both conditions are aggravated by the repetitive wrist movements, specifically hammering, rowing, and racquet sports.

9. **Undisplaced fracture and osteonecrosis**—easily identifiable with severe pain, swelling, and deformity. Such fractures are managed acutely based on the degree of displacement and involvement of joint. Nondisplaced fracture or stress fracture can be missed because of false-negative initial x-ray results and lack of significant history of trauma. In patients with high-risk factors, such as osteoporosis and mineral bone disease, minor trauma or repetitive overuse can lead to fracture. Examination typically reveals discreet and subtle tenderness at the site of fracture. High level of suspicion is required for patients with risk factors. In young athletes engaged in repetitive compressive impact and torsion forces, epiphyseal injury known as gymnast wrist should also be suspected.[7] Missed or unhealing fracture can cause osteonecrosis of carpal bones, commonly in scaphoid and lunate. In addition, avascular necrosis can also occur in carpal bones (Kienbock disease involving lunate) with insidious onset of pain, swelling, and decreased wrist ROM.[8]

10. **Benign and malignant tumor**—rare in the hand and wrist, accounting for 6% of bony tumors[9] or metastasis; however, tumor should be included in the differential diagnosis for patients with a history of cancer or red flags. Most tumors in the hand are benign, with giant cell tumor of the tendon sheath being the most common. Giant cell tumors are typically located in the distal radius and middle phalanx and radial three digits.[10] Although some cases are asymptomatic, presentation is usually progressive worsening of pain, which eventually becomes constant. Pain is often worse at night or with rest. Systemic manifestation such as weight loss is uncommon.

11. **Osteomyelitis or septic arthritis**—similar to malignancy, red flags such as trauma, open/puncture/bite wound, history of acquired immunodeficiency syndrome (AIDS), intravenous drug abuse, and poorly controlled diabetes should increase suspicion for infection.[11] With persistent wound or cellulitis, osteomyelitis or septic arthritis should be strongly considered. There is constant pain, often without any systemic symptoms. Infection may present with redness, warmth (increased temperature), and/or subtle swelling. C-reactive protein (CRP) and erythrocyte sedimentation rate (ESR) are frequently elevated, although white blood cell count may be normal.

12. **Referred pain from cervical spine and elbow**—typically presents with neck and elbow pain in addition to hand/wrist pain. The patient describes radiating pain from the neck down to the hand. Cervical radiculopathy (C6–C8) presents with neck pain radiating down to the forearm and distally to the fingers. C7 radiculopathy, the most common level, presents with neck pain radiating down to the hand and fingers, particularly to third digit. C6 radiculopathy radiates to the thumb and index finger, and to the ring and little finger in C8 radiculopathy. Spurling test can be specific if it reproduces radiating pain down to the hand (sensitivity 30%–60% and specificity 92%–100%).[12,13] The elbow is an underrecognized pain generator. Posterior interosseous nerve entrapment syndrome may cause deep wrist pain lacking typical sensory symptoms without elbow pain in many cases.

13. **Other neuropathic pain**—complex regional pain syndrome (CRPS) present with pain in the hand, as well as in the shoulder (shoulder-hand syndrome). CRPS may occur after nerve injury (type 2) or following minor injury, without a specific nerve injury (type 1). There is spontaneous pain, hyperalgesia/allodynia beyond the distribution of single nerve or root that is disproportionate to the inciting event. Trophic changes, such as hypertrophic nails, disturbance of hair growth, atrophic skin, edema, sudomotor abnormalities (dry, warm, erythematous extremity, cold or hyperhidrosis) may be appreciated on examination. Early recognition and aggressive management is important. Cutaneous neuropathy, such as Wartenberg syndrome from superficial radial neuropathy presents with pain, tingling, pins/needle sensation in the radial side of the wrist and hand. The pain and sensory symptoms may radiate proximally toward the elbow. Careful palpation of the lesion to trigger or reproduce the symptom (Valleix phenomenon) is a useful physical examination technique.

Case Discussion

Absence of pain in the proximal upper extremity or neck makes referred or radiating pain less likely. Local wrist and hand pain can be divided into neuropathic, musculoskeletal, or combined.

Presence of positive sensory symptom (tingling paresthesia) in this case suggests neuropathic pain generators. Localization of the symptom into the hand and wrist makes a focal entrapment neuropathy more likely over cervical radiculopathy, brachial plexopathy, complex regional pain syndrome, or others.

Location of sensory symptoms and signs is very useful in differentiating peripheral entrapment syndrome in most cases. For example, symptoms in the palmar-radial aspect suggest carpal tunnel syndrome, ulnar side symptoms suggest ulnar neuropathy, and dorsal-radial symptoms suggest sensory radial neuropathy. As in this case, patients often have difficulty describing the exact location of sensory symptoms. In addition, there are musculoskeletal mimickers with positive sensory symptoms. Coexisting musculoskeletal pathology and focal entrapment syndrome are not uncommon.

Musculoskeletal pain generators in the radial aspect of the wrist include pathologies involving radiocarpal, scaphotrapezial, trapeziometacarpal, scaphoid-trapezium-trapezoid, scapholunate joints, ligaments, first dorsal extensor column (APL, EPB), and extensor pollicis longus.

Systematic palpation of structures is useful in delineating local pathologies. Provocative maneuvers can be applied to different structures. CMC grind test (rotation of the first metacarpal while axial loading) can reproduce pain from CMC joint while stretching by ulnar deviation can aggravate symptoms from de Quervain tenosynovitis. Resisted contraction of muscle (without joint movement) can also help to differentiate pain from joint structure or tendon/tenosynovium.

Shifting the scaphoid while pressing the distal pole of the scaphoid (pressure toward the dorsum) during radioulnar deviation of the wrist (scaphoid shift test) can reproduce the symptom mediated by scapholunate instability.

Pain reproduced by supination from pronation in an ulnarly deviated wrist is specific for ulnar triquetral impaction syndrome as the supination decreases the space between the ulnar and triquetrum.

Differential palpation can also be useful. Tenderness on the distal scaphoid tubercle at the level of distal wrist crease may suggest scaphoid bony pathology. The scaphotrapezial joint is located immediately distal to the distal pole of the scaphoid (see Fig. 5.2). The trapezium-first metacarpal joint is easily palpated from the proximal end of the first metacarpal, as it is located more radially and has a shape similar to the shoulder.

The pisiform is located at the ulnar side of distal wrist crease, opposite to the distal pole of scaphoid. Tenderness of the pisiform may indicate FCU enthesopathy or pisotriquetral arthropathy. Grinding of the pisiform (movement with compression) can reproduce pain on the pisiform versus worsening pain on resisted wrist flexion and ulnar deviation favoring FCU tendinopathy. Palpation of the fovea located immediately distal to the ulnar styloid process can be useful for TFCC lesion.

Paresthesia indicates the involvement of sensory nerve pathways, but often not specific in terms of size of nerve fibers. Pins/needle sensation, burning can suggest involvement of small fibers whereas loss of proprioception and light touch indicates large fiber involvement.

Electrodiagnosis (EMG) test can be particularly useful to evaluate subclinical/mild motor deficit or symptoms from large sensory fibers. In addition to localizing the lesion, EMG can characterize the lesion into axonal, demyelinating, or mixed lesions, which can guide treatment and provide severity and prognosis. In this case, an EMG test to evaluate paresthesias may be useful.

Absence of red flags, in this case, lowers the possibilities of infections or malignancy as the underlying cause although cannot be completely excluded. If there is any concern, imaging (at least x-ray), and laboratory tests should be done (ESR and CRP) to evaluate these possibilities.

Objective Data

Complete blood count—within normal limits
Complete metabolic panel—within normal limits
X-ray of wrist and hand—calcification in the TFCC. Decreased joint space in the first metacarpal-trapezium joint. No fracture or dislocation. No sclerotic or lytic lesions.
Nerve conduction study and needle EMG was negative
ESR and CRP—within normal limits
Additional serologic test (rheumatoid factor, anticyclic citrullinated peptide antibody, antinuclear antibody, uric acid)—within normal limits

Case Discussion

Laboratory test and imaging studies are often unnecessary for initial management of common musculoskeletal conditions. However, imaging may be useful in the presence of red flags or unsatisfactory response to initial conservative management. Imaging is indicated in cases of preceding trauma, especially in persons with risk factors for fracture. Imaging is required if there was significant trauma, chronic pain despite conservative treatment, or progressive nature of presentation. Blood work and imaging are very useful if there are specific indications for each study based on clinical impressions.

In this case, the laboratory and imaging data are helpful to further narrow down the differential diagnosis. Advanced imaging, such as MRI, is required if an initial x-ray fails to reveal any pathology despite persistent pain after preceding injury or trauma to evaluate intramedullary pathology, chronic osteonecrosis, and soft tissue pathology. MRI is the gold standard imaging modality in chronic wrist and hand pain with a high level of sensitivity. However, findings may not always correlate with clinical presentation. Therefore it is important to interpret abnormal imaging findings based on the patient's symptoms and signs. Other limitations include high cost, limited access, and inability to evaluate dynamically (in conventional settings). Evaluation of intraarticular pathology often requires MRI arthrogram, which has a higher sensitivity. Computed tomography (CT) is less commonly used, in part because of limited capacity to evaluate soft tissues. CT can be useful in the evaluation of fractures and preoperative planning.

With the increasing availability of musculoskeletal ultrasound (US) in outpatient settings, the utility of point-of-care US in hand and wrist disorders has expanded beyond a tool for guiding injections. US can be particularly useful in evaluating soft tissue pathologies such as tendon/tenosynovium, superficial joint/synovial, ligamentous, and peripheral nerves.

In this patient, the lack of ulnar-sided wrist pain makes calcification in TFCC less likely as a generator of pain. Calcification in the TFCC complex may occur in degenerative processes or chondrocalcinosis.

X-ray of this patient revealed typical findings suggesting degenerative changes involving trapezium-first metacarpal joint, the most common location for OA in the hand and wrist. Without red flags and any lytic or blastic lesions on x-ray, bony tumor or metastatic disease would be unlikely, although plain x-ray can miss mild or early disease or lesions. Infection can be eliminated as a cause based on absence of red flags and normal ESR and CRP levels.

Nerve conduction study (NCS) and needle EMG test are sensitive and specific for focal entrapment neuropathies in the wrist. Therefore negative findings are sufficient to rule out focal entrapment neuropathies as the underlying etiology for tingling paresthesias. Note that NCS is limited in evaluating small fiber lesions, and needle EMG is limited in evaluating mild cervical radiculopathy, unless axonal and motor segment of the nerve root is involved. Clinically, cervical radiculopathy was low on the differential diagnosis in this case because the patient did not present with any neck pain, radiating arm pain, motor or sensory deficit in specific root distribution.

Review of Proposed Pathology and Pathobiomechanics in Carpometacarpal Joint

Trapezium-first metacarpal (first CMC) joint is a saddle joint that lacks osseous stability, allowing freedom of movement while being stabilized by multiple ligaments. The saddle joint structure allows three arcs of motion: abduction-adduction (perpendicular to the palmar plane), flexion-extension (parallel to the palmar plane), opposition (flexion and abduction)-reposition. Among ligament stabilizers, oblique beak ligament and dorsoradial ligament are the most important stabilizers, primarily restraining dorsoradial subluxation (Fig. 5.3).

Opposition requires axial rotation with increased contact forces in the first CMC joint. Flexion-adduction also increases compressive force of the joint, particularly at the volar articular surface.

Lateral pinch of thumb and index finger increases joint compressive force by 12 times. Repetitive thumb pinches can increase the risk of developing symptomatic joint disease. Excessive laxity of the joint with repetitive loading may lead to inflammation with synovitis, while shear forces contribute to wear pattern and joint narrowing. Osteophytes and dorsoradial subluxation

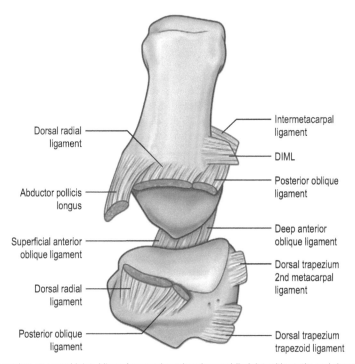

Dorsal radial ligament

Intermetacarpal ligament

DIML

Posterior oblique ligament

Abductor pollicis longus

Superficial anterior oblique ligament

Deep anterior oblique ligament

Dorsal trapezium 2nd metacarpal ligament

Dorsal radial ligament

Posterior oblique ligament

Dorsal trapezium trapezoid ligament

Fig. 5.3 Trapeziometacarpal joint. Hinged open view showing saddle joint with static and dynamic stabilizers, superficial, deep anterior oblique ligament, cut dorsoradial ligament, posterior oblique ligament, and abductor pollicis long. *DIML*, Dorsal intermetacarpal ligament. (From P.M. Fox, B.T. Carlsen, S.L. Moran. Osteoarthritis in the hand and wrist, In: Plastic Surgery: Hand and Upper Extremity, vol 6, 4e, Elsevier, London, 2018, 440–477.)

of first metacarpal bone can occur. This subluxation of the base of the metacarpal bone with unopposed action of the adductor pollicis muscle leads to progressive deficit of grip strength (e.g., during spreading the hand around the jar).

As high as 43% of patients with CMC arthritis have coexisting carpal tunnel syndrome. Although the exact mechanism is unknown, previous studies suggest the synovitis involved in CMC arthritis may extend to flexor tenosynovium.[14] Alterations in the peritrapezial anatomy affect intracarpal tunnel pressure, as the transcarpal ligament attaches to the trapezial ridge.[15]

CLINICAL SIGNS AND SYMPTOMS OF OSTEOARTHRITIS OF TRAPEZIO-FIRST METACARPAL JOINT ARTHROPATHY

Patients present with insidious radial-sided hand and thumb pain. Pain is aggravated by handwriting, holding, turning doorknobs, and using scissors. Functional limitations vary depending on the patient's vocation and avocations.

Pain can vary from intermittent dull ache to persistent sharp pain. In advanced stages, pain may not be localized to the joint. There may be mild weakness of thumb secondary to pain.

In isolated OA, neurologic examination will be negative other than mild weakness in the thumb, particularly opposition (abduction and flexion). However, muscle strength is also affected by concomitant peripheral entrapment neuropathy, especially carpal tunnel syndrome, or tendon tear.

TABLE 5.2 ■ Common X-ray Findings of Wrist and Hand Pathologies

Osteoarthritis	Joint space narrowing, osteophytes, subchondral sclerosis, and cystic change
Rheumatoid arthritis	Juxtaarticular osteopenia, marginal erosions, joint space narrowing, subluxation, and periarticular soft tissue swelling
Gout	Juxtaarticular erosions with a "punched-out" appearance, sclerotic borders, overhanging edges, and soft-tissue tophi
Calcium crystal deposition disease	Calcium crystal deposition in the soft tissues (joint cartilage and triangular fibrous cartilage complex) Joint space narrowing, osteophytes, and subchondral cysts in a distribution that is not typical for osteoarthritis (e.g., metacarpophalangeal joints)
Psoriatic arthritis	Pencil-in-cup deformity (expansion of the base of the distal phalanx with destruction of the head of the middle phalanx), acroosteolysis, and whole-digit soft tissue swelling ("sausage digit")
Lupus arthropathy	Joint subluxations without erosions, joint space narrowing, periarticular osteoporosis
Septic arthropathy	Initially: normal x-ray imaging, or periarticular soft tissue swelling and/or joint space widening with effusion With progression: joint space narrowing, poorly defined erosions, and marginal erosions as uncovered intracapsular bone is destroyed
Neuropathic joint	Initially: normal x-ray imaging With progression (which can be very rapid): severe cartilage loss, fragmentation of subchondral bone with pathological fracture → disintegration of joint structure and juxtaarticular cortical bone loss

(From S.W. Lee, Musculoskeletal Injuries and Conditions: Assessment and Management. Demos Medical, New York, 2017.)

Particular attention to the presence of splitting sensation in the fourth digit (present in focal median nerve entrapment neuropathy) and sparing of sensation in the thenar eminence (innervated by palmar cutaneous nerve coursing superficial to the transcarpal ligament) is necessary.

Deep tendon reflexes are normal unless there is coexisting peripheral nerve lesion or upper motor neuron lesion. Loss of deep tendon reflexes are particularly useful for diagnosing cervical radiculopathy. Hoffman sign is negative unless there is concomitant upper motor neuron disorder, such as cervical myelopathy, motor neuron diseases, or multiple sclerosis.

IMAGING STUDIES

Plain x-ray is very useful in identifying degenerative joint disease versus other arthropathy, such as RA or crystal deposition disease (Table 5.2). Typical radiographs of the thumb include three views: anterior-posterior, lateral, and oblique views. There are different views for specific anatomy, such as the basal-joint stress view to assess degree of trapezio-metacarpal subluxation and the lateral pinch view (axial loading by pinching) to quantify basal joint height.[16] These extra views are typically obtained for surgical planning or postoperative follow-up. Several image-based classification systems are available. Criteria suggested by Eaton and Littler is widely used, with stage I having normal articular cartilage and a widened joint space to stage IV having significant first CMC joint deterioration with concomitant scaphotrapezial joint degeneration.[17]

US is an easily accessible tool that can be used during the initial evaluation. In busy clinics, point-of-care US can be used to confirm diagnosis and evaluate differential diagnoses. US is particularly useful for evaluating soft tissues, joint effusions, osteophytes, and chondrocalcinosis in the CMC and neighboring joints. US can also show focal nerve entrapment, such as carpal tunnel syndrome or tenosynovitis (e.g., de Quervain tenosynovitis).[18]

DISCUSSION

Two distinctive elements of differential diagnoses should be considered. One must rule out inflammatory (rheumatologic) conditions and infectious conditions, such as osteomyelitis. Systemic features beyond the unilateral hand and wrist, red flags such as fever, chills, history of cancer should always be investigated further.

Inflammatory arthropathy, especially RA, should be recognized as early systemic treatment and is required to slow down disease progress. RA can be ruled out with lack of systemic features, negative serologic tests (negative rheumatoid factor, anticyclic citrullinated peptide antibody, antinuclear antibody), and negative imaging tests.

Degree of radiologic advancement can assist in prognostication. Conservative management is strongly advocated in this patient as first-line treatment. Although there is limited research available, most authors agree nonoperative treatment is effective in first CMC OA. A multimodal approach is highly advocated consisting of occupational therapy, splinting, pharmacotherapy, and surgical referral if high-quality conservative management fails.

ACUTE PHASE

In the inflammatory phase, a short course of antiinflammatory (either over the counter [OTC] or prescribed) may be beneficial. An OTC patch or cream (salicylate, lidocaine, or capsaicin) may be used to decrease pain. An OTC thumb spica splint used at night or at rest can help relieve symptoms. Often a cock-up splint is prescribed or purchased by the patient, which may aggravate symptoms by creating more motion in the first CMC joint, by limiting movement of neighboring joints, such as the wrist. Education to modify the provoking activity is necessary.

A short course of acetaminophen and nonsteroidal antiinflammatory drugs (NSAIDs) can help manage pain. The risks of taking NSAIDs in those with cardiovascular, renal, and gastrointestinal disease should be reviewed.

Tramadol, a weak opioid analgesic, has been considered as a potential alternative to NSAIDs because of lower cardiovascular and gastrointestinal risk. Prescribers should be aware that tramadol may be associated with increased risk for mortality in patients with OA.[19]

Strong narcotic analgesics, muscle relaxants, antidepressants, and anticonvulsants are rarely used in hand OA. Long-term use of opioid analgesics should be avoided.

Occupational or Physical Therapy

Referral to occupational therapy (or hand therapy) program to evaluate activities of daily living (ADL), instrumental ADL, adaptive equipment, restore ROM, taping, joint mobilization, neurodynamic therapy, fabrication of orthoses, strengthening exercise of hand muscles should be considered. Modalities, including heat, electrical stimulation, and US, are useful temporary modulators of pain. Precautions should be taken to prevent cold-or heat-related injury. Gradual strengthening program follows once pain relief and full ROM are achieved. Some isometric strengthening exercises can be engaged even before full ROM is achieved. A systematic review demonstrated resistance strengthening exercises were effective on mild joint pain relief but not on hand function or grip strength.[20] Multimodal therapy is shown to be more effective than unimodal therapy for patients with first CMC OA.[21]

Injections

Intraarticular steroid injection with/without US guidance can help relieve pain. Short- and long-term benefits of intraarticular steroid injections were mixed, from no benefit over placebo to lasting benefits up to 12 months follow-up. Other injections include hyaluronic acid with possibly superior pain relief after 6 months over steroid injections.[22] There is limited evidence for platelet-rich plasma injection to the CMC joint.

Referral to Surgery

If a patient fails to respond to nonoperative therapy after at least a 6-month period with disabling pain and decreased function, referral to hand surgery can be considered. Surgical interventions include ligament reconstruction with tendon slip and tendon interposition, arthroscopy, complete trapezium resection, abduction-extension osteotomy, or total joint arthroplasty. Cochrane review failed to demonstrate any superior techniques over another in pain and function.[27,28] Further details of each surgical technique is beyond the scope of this chapter. Postoperative rehabilitation focuses on gaining abduction initially.

Summary

A patient presents with chronic dominant-side hand and wrist pain, worsening over time, without involvement of other joints or red flags, equivocal sensory symptoms, and demonstrable clinical signs, including positive CMC grind test. Because of the chronicity of the pain, imaging study was ordered, and EMG was done to evaluate sensory symptoms. X-ray findings with the clinical presentation were consistent with OA involving first CMC joint, and the stage based on x-ray findings was early.

She received pain management with OTC NSAIDS, acetaminophen, OTC thumb spica splint, and educated on activity modification to decrease risk factors. At 6 weeks follow-up, there is some improvement but she still complains of significant pain. Intraarticular steroid injection was done, followed by a short course of occupational therapy. Occupational therapy consisted of joint mobilization, gradual resistive strengthening exercise of the thenar and extrinsic thumb muscles, fabrication of long thumb spica splint with Thermo moldable materials, instrumental ADL exercise, adaptive equipment evaluation, education of biomechanics, and home exercise program. She responded favorably to these regiments. At a follow-up visit 3 months later, the patient remained pain-free and improved in her daily activities. She continues to remain on a home exercise program.

Key Points

- Patients with hand and wrist pain should be carefully assessed using a systematic approach. Different approaches are available, based on the characteristic or location of the pain.
- A focused history and physical examination can lead to accurate clinical diagnosis with confirmation through imaging, serologic test, and electromyography.
- Most disorders of the hand and wrist respond favorably to conservative management, especially with the correct diagnosis and approach.

CLINICAL PEARLS

Trapezium-first metacarpal (carpometacarpal [CMC]) joint is a saddle joint that allows three arcs of motion: abduction-adduction (perpendicular to the palmar plane), flexion-extension (parallel to the palmar plane), opposition (flexion and abduction)-reposition.

Common musculoskeletal pain generators in the radial aspect of the wrist and hand include arthropathies of first CMC joint, metacarpophalangeal joint, scapholunate ligament injury, and de Quervain disease.

Multimodal therapies, including thumb spica brace, strengthening exercise, adaptive equipment, and activity modification, can be useful treatment for first CMC arthropathy.

References

1. J.M. Daniels 2nd, E.G. Zook, J.M. Lynch, Hand and wrist injuries: Part II. Emergent evaluation, Am. Fam. Physician 69 (8) (2004) 1949–1956.
2. J. Yao, M.J. Park, Early treatment of degenerative arthritis of the thumb carpometacarpal joint, Hand Clin. 24 (3) (2008) 251–261, v–vi.
3. J.S. Smolen, D. Aletaha, I.B. McInnes, Rheumatoid arthritis, Lancet 388 (10055) (2016) 2023–2038.
4. D. Aletaha, T. Neogi, A.J. Silman, et al., Rheumatoid arthritis classification criteria: an American College of Rheumatology/European League Against Rheumatism collaborative initiative, Arthritis Rheum. 62 (9) (2010) 2569–2581.
5. C.T. Ritchlin, R.A. Colbert, D.D. Gladman, Psoriatic arthritis, N. Engl. J. Med. 376 (10) (2017) 957–970.
6. M.S. Day, D. Nam, S. Goodman, E.P. Su, M. Figgie, Psoriatic arthritis, J. Am. Acad. Orthop. Surg. 20 (1) (2012) 28–37.
7. H.J. Benjamin, S.C. Engel, D. Chudzik, Wrist pain in gymnasts: a review of common overuse wrist pathology in the gymnastics athlete, Curr. Sports Med. Rep. 16 (5) (2017) 322–329.
8. D. Cross, K.S. Matullo, Kienbock disease, Orthop. Clin. North Am. 45 (1) (2014) 141–152.
9. M.J. Simon, P. Pogoda, F. Hövelborn, et al., Incidence, histopathologic analysis and distribution of tumours of the hand, BMC Musculoskelet Disord 15 (2014) 182.
10. W.D. Middleton, V. Patel, S.A. Teefey, M.I. Boyer, Giant cell tumors of the tendon sheath: analysis of sonographic findings, AJR Am. J. Roentgenol. 183 (2) (2004) 337–339.
11. O.I. Franko, R.A. Abrams, Hand infections, Orthop. Clin. North Am. 44 (4) (2013) 625–634.
12. H.C. Tong, A.J. Haig, K. Yamakawa, The Spurling test and cervical radiculopathy, Spine 27 (2) (2002) 156–159.
13. S. Shabat, Y. Leitner, R. David, Y. Folman, The correlation between Spurling test and imaging studies in detecting cervical radiculopathy, J. Neuroimaging 22 (4) (2012) 375–378.
14. C.P. Melone Jr., B. Beavers, A. Isani, The basal joint pain syndrome, Clin. Orthop. Relat. Res. 220 (1987) 58–67.
15. K. Lutsky, A. Ilyas, N. Kim, P. Beredjiklian, Basal joint arthroplasty decreases carpal tunnel pressure, Hand (N Y), 10 (3) (2015) 403–406.
16. O.A. Barron, S.Z. Glickel, R.G. Eaton, Basal joint arthritis of the thumb, J. Am. Acad. Orthop. Surg. 8 (5) (2000) 314–323.
17. A.E. Van Heest, P. Kallemeier, Thumb carpal metacarpal arthritis, J. Am. Acad. Orthop. Surg. 16 (3) (2008) 140–151.
18. D.M. Melville, M.S. Taljanovic, L.R. Scalcione, et al., Imaging and management of thumb carpometacarpal joint osteoarthritis, Skeletal Radiol. 44 (2) (2015) 165–177.
19. C. Zeng, M. Dubreuil, M.R. LaRochelle, Association of tramadol with all-cause mortality among patients with osteoarthritis, J. Am. Med. Assoc. 321 (10) (2019) 969–982.
20. N.E. Magni, P.J. McNair, D.A. Rice, The effects of resistance training on muscle strength, joint pain, and hand function in individuals with hand osteoarthritis: a systematic review and meta-analysis, Arthritis Res. Ther. 19 (1) (2017) 131.
21. M. Ahern, J. Skyllas, A. Wajon, J. Hush, The effectiveness of physical therapies for patients with base of thumb osteoarthritis: systematic review and meta-analysis, Musculoskelet. Sci. Pract. 35 (2018) 46–54.
22. S. Fuchs, R. Mönikes, A. Wohlmeiner, T. Heyse, Intra-articular hyaluronic acid compared with corticoid injections for the treatment of rhizarthrosis, Osteoarthritis Cartilage 14 (1) (2006) 82–88.
23. R. Shereen, M. Loukas, R.S. Tubbs, Extensor digitorum brevis manus: a comprehensive review of this variant muscle of the dorsal hand, Cureus 9 (8) (2017) e1568–e1568.
24. S. Badhe, J. Lynch, S.K. Thorpe, L.C. Bainbridge, Operative treatment of Linburg-Comstock syndrome, J. Bone. Joint. Surg. Br. 92 (9) (2010) 1278–1281.
25. P. Saffar, Chondrocalcinosis of the wrist, J. Hand Surg. Br. 29 (5) (2004) 486–493.
26. A.K. Rosenthal, L.M. Ryan, Calcium pyrophosphate deposition disease, N. Engl. J. Med. 374 (26) (2016) 2575–2584.
27. A. Wajon, T. Vinycomb, E. Carr, I. Edmunds, L. Ada, Surgery for thumb (trapeziometacarpal joint) osteoarthritis, Cochrane Database Syst. Rev. 2015 (2) (2015) CD004631.
28. G.M. Vermeulen, H. Slijper, R. Feitz, S.E. Hovius, T.M. Moojen, R.W. Selles, Surgical management of primary thumb carpometacarpal osteoarthritis: a systematic review, J. Hand. Surg. Am. 36 (1) (2011) 157–169.

CHAPTER 6

Hip Pain

Dr. Se Won Lee, MD ▪ Dr. Patrick Mahaney, MD, MS, FAAPMR

Case Presentation

A 32-year-old man presents to the Physical Medicine and Rehabilitation (PM&R) clinic with right hip pain. He describes that the pain is gradually worsening over the last 3 months and located deep in the groin. He has had intermittent groin pain for more than 1 year and denies any preceding injury or trauma. The pain is worse with prolonged walking and playing soccer in the weekend. He stopped playing soccer 2 months ago. He takes over-the-counter acetaminophen and ibuprofen with temporary relief. There is intermittent posterior thigh pain in the right side as well. He reports his sleep is disturbed because of this pain. He denies numbness, tingling, focal weakness, "giving way" sensation, or recurrent falls. He reports intermittent knee pain in the right side and intermittent midline lower lumbar pain. He was referred by his primary care doctor.

Past medical history: He denies any significant past medical history, including hypertension, diabetes, increased cholesterol, developmental delays, or pediatric orthopedic conditions.

Social history: He works as a civil servant, lives with wife in 3rd-floor apartment with elevator. He continues to jog (about 20 miles per week) in the community park but stopped playing soccer during weekend because of pain.

Past surgical history: None

Allergies: No known drug allergy

Medications: Occasional ibuprofen 400 mg

BP: 130/76 mmHg, RR: 16/min, PR: 75 per min, Temp: 97° F, Ht: 5'8", Wt: 164 lbs, BMI: 24.9 kg/m^2

General: Well built, not in acute distress. He is alert and oriented to person, place, and time.

Extremities: No edema, no skin rashes, no erythema, no surgical scars, no open wound.

NEUROMUSCULOSKELETAL EXAMINATION

Inspection of lower extremity: No gross deformity. No gross muscle atrophy.

Range of motion of lumbar spine: Within functional limits.

Motor exam: 5/5 symmetrically except right hip flexion, and extension which is pain limited to 5–/5.

Deep tendon reflexes: 2+ in quadriceps femoris and triceps surae bilaterally.

Sensory exam: Intact to light touch and pinprick in all dermatomes of both lower extremities.

Tone: Normal

Gait: Antalgic

Provocation tests

Straight leg raise test: Negative

Slump test: Negative

Patrick (flexion, abduction, and external rotation) test: Reproducing groin pain.

Pace maneuver (for piriformis syndrome): Negative.

Flexion, adduction, and internal rotation (FAIR): Pain in the groin.

Ely test: Tight rectus femoris in the right side.

Modified Thomas test: No significant hip flexion contracture noted. Symmetric.

No tenderness on the greater trochanter.

Posterior superior iliac spine: Not tender.

General Discussion: General Approach to Hip Pain

The initial focus should be to differentiate local musculoskeletal conditions, such as intra- or extraarticular hip joint complex pathologies and also from other referred pain generators, such as lumbar spine or sacroiliac joint pathologies. Although both conditions coexist frequently, it is better to identify the primary or predominant pain generator for effective management.

The demographic information, such as age, gender, and detailed information of the groin pain (particularly the location of pain, mechanism of injury, aggravating and relieving factor) can be useful in narrowing down the differential diagnoses. Review of system and past medical history also provide valuable information.

Local musculoskeletal pathologies can be grouped based on the location of the pain, as illustrated in Table 6.1. In this table, the groin region was divided based on the groin triangle, defined by anterior superior iliac spine, pubic tubercle, and midline between the anterior superior iliac spine and superior pole of the patellar.[1] Characteristics of the pain can be useful to differentiate the neuropathic versus musculoskeletal (nociceptive) pain. This patient does not have typical radiating pain from the lower back to the groin nor sensory symptoms, favoring the local musculoskeletal pathologies for pain generator. The young age of the patient argues against degenerative osteoarthritis (OA); however, it cannot be ruled out.

The physical examination can focus on the neuromuscular examination, including inspection for atrophy of muscles, evaluation of focal motor (weakness of muscle with/without deformity [indicating chronic imbalance of muscle strength]) or sensory deficit (sensation to large fiber mediated light touch and proprioception and small-fiber mediated pinprick and temperature sensation) in each dermatome or peripheral nerve distribution, as well as deep tendon reflexes.

TABLE 6.1 ■ **Local Hip Pathologies Based on the Location of Pain and Maximal Tenderness**

Location	Pathologies and Characteristics
Superior	Rectus abdominis insertional tendinopathy Sportsman hernia
Lateral	Femoral neck fracture: pain on internal rotation/hopping, often significant trauma history missing in osteoporotic elderly or stress fracture with underlying risk factors
	Trochanteric bursitis, gluteal tendinopathy/tear, proximal iliotibial band syndrome and Morel-Lavallee lesion
	Meralgia paresthetica; with minor trauma/irritation (e.g., belt or weight loss or gain)
Medial (pubic tubercle)	Pubic bone stress injury (osteitis pubis), degenerative pubic symphysis: worsening pain with stair climbing
	Inferior ramus bony injury (including stress fracture): worse with hopping Rectus abdominis enthesopathy
	Adductor/gracilis avulsion/enthesopathy/tendinopathy at musculotendinous junction[30]
	External iliac A endofibrosis: reproducible thigh discomfort after high-intensity exercise (e.g., cycling)
In groin triangle	Iliopsoas tendinopathy/tear, iliopectineal bursitis
	Rectus femoris calcific tendonitis, musculotendinous junction tear
	Hip osteoarthritis Femoroacetabular impingement/labral pathology: younger adults Slipped femoral epiphysis: in adolescents Avascular necrosis with medical comorbidities and Legg-Calve-Perthes disease (children aged <12 years)
	Genitofemoral and medial femoral cutaneous nerve lesion: neuropathic pain Femoral hernia: painful lump inferomedial to pubic tubercle

(From S.W. Lee, Musculoskeletal Injuries and Conditions: Assessment and Management, Demos Medical, New York, 2017; N.E. Magni, P.J. McNair, D.A. Rice, The effects of resistance training on muscle strength, joint pain, and hand function in individuals with hand osteoarthritis: a systematic review and meta-analysis, Arthritis Res. Ther. 19 (1) (2017) 131.)

Focal neurologic deficit in the groin region can be explained by pathologies involving lumbar roots (L1–3), lumbar plexus, and its branches, such as iliohypogastric, ilioinguinal, genitofemoral mononeuropathies, or pathologies involving muscles (myopathy, polymyalgia rheumatica, possibly pelvic floor dysfunction with functional deficit). Occasionally, referred pain from musculoskeletal pathologies (e.g., facet joint mediated pain or myofascial pain syndrome) can be perceived as positive sensory symptoms.

Common Differential Diagnoses for Hip Pain

1. **Hip osteoarthritis**—OA of the hip joint is common especially in the older population with prevalence of radiographic findings of hip OA up to 27%.[2] It is more common in females than males, Caucsians and African Americans. The pain from OA is often vague, most commonly in the groin but can be around the hip joint (anterior, lateral, and posterior aspect [buttock pain, up to 71% of people with hip OA]) possibly with referred leg pain.[3,4] The onset of pain is usually insidious without any preceding injury or trauma and frequently accompanied by morning stiffness (<1 hour). The pain is aggravated by prolonged standing, walking, stair negotiation, or any prolonged weight-bearing activity. However, this is not specific to OA

2. **Femoroacetabular impingement**—a problem among active younger and middle age population, hip (femoroacetabular) joint impingement secondary to abnormal morphology (femoral head-neck junction and/or acetabulum). Because there is high prevalence of these morphological abnormalities among asymptomatic young population, it is often challenging to correlate this abnormal morphology to patient's symptom. The presentation seems to be similar to hip OA with groin pain and buttock pain, but can be in the lower back, anterior thigh, and knee pain. The "C-sign," forming the letter C with one's hand with the index at the anterior superior iliac spine (ASIS) and thumb toward the posterior superior iliac spine (PSIS) with the palm over the lateral hip on description of the location of the pain is historically classic for femoral acetabular joint pathology (such as impingement syndrome) but the overall diagnostic utility of this sign/aspect of the history is questionable.[5] There are often concomitant (or secondary to femoroacetabular impingement) pathologies, such as labral tear or chondral defect/delamination seen on advanced imaging that can complicate the picture. Activities requiring flexion of the hip (crouching or sitting) or athletic activities are limited with pain. The symptoms can be reproduced by impingement position, such as flexion, adduction, and internal rotation (FADIR) of the hip joint.[6]

3. **Inflammatory arthropathies**—presents with groin, trochanteric, and/or buttock pain, often associated with prolonged stiffness. The pain often gets better with activity. Multiple/bilateral joint involvement, fatigue, and other systemic symptoms are common. There is a variation of hip joint involvement between different inflammatory arthropathies. For example, ankylosing spondylosis commonly involves hip joint (<50%) with lower back/buttock pain, but psoriatic arthropathy and gout rarely affects the hip joint.[7]

4. **Labral tear**—can be present on advanced imaging without any symptoms, therefore it is often difficult to correlate the imaging finding to the patient's presentation. Reproduction of symptoms with the impingement of the specifically located labrum in the context of the relevant history is supportive of the labral tear as the pain generator. Response from diagnostic hip joint injection can be helpful as well. Most susceptible location is the anterosuperior labrum because of stress during hip flexion and internal rotation frequently happening during pivoting activities. Patient may present with "pop" along with catching sensation, pain in the groin or buttock depending on the location of the labrum.[8]

5. **Avascular necrosis**—if there are risk factors, such as history of trauma, radiation, sickle cell disease, steroid use, alcohol abuse, and so on, avascular necrosis should be included

in differential diagnosis. Peak incidence is between second to fifth decades of life (most common in mid-30s), more common in males than females (varies depending on studies with equivalence in gender prevalence in some studies), and often bilateral (40%–80%).[9] Pain is often insidious at onset, gradually worsening, and becomes constant eventually. Weight-bearing activity and range of motion (ROM) of the hip joint (particularly internal rotation) can be painful with limitation. As the presentation is similar to other hip joint pathologies, a high index of suspicion is required and this can often be obtained from the risk factors elicited in the history. This allows for the appropriate imaging study to be ordered for diagnosis. One should remember that early stages of avascular necrosis (without femoral head collapse) can be missed on plain radiographs (with sensitivity as low as 41%).[10]

6. **Strains and sprain**—if there was a preceding trauma and injury, strains and sprains can be suspected for the underlying etiology after fracture is ruled out. Frequently, the imaging studies are negative other than avulsion injury at the insertion site. Depending on the mechanism of injury and location of pain, the localization of the muscle injury can be easily done if the time is taken to isolate the various muscles about the hip much in the same way one does with the rotator cuff in the shoulder. In significant muscle strains or tear, ecchymosis can occur. Examination can be nonspecific but tenderness and reproduction of symptoms with muscle/tendon/ligament stretching (or resistive strengthening) can help to identify the lesion. Typically, there is no neurologic symptom other than irritation of cutaneous nerve (by overlying/neighboring tendon or ligament).

7. **Trochanteric bursitis (greater trochanteric pain syndrome)**—one of the most common sources of pain in the hip, prevalence up to 5.6 per 1000, more common in females than males, and peak incidence in fourth to sixth decades. Bursitis can occur with/without any preceding injury or trauma. Other risk factors include leg-length discrepancy, pelvic obliquity, running on banked surface, and obesity.[11] The pain is typically located in the slightly posterior aspect of the greater trochanter (where subgluteus maximus bursa located). A gluteus medius tendinopathy, tear, or avulsion may produce point tenderness in a similar area. The patient often complains of difficulty sleeping on the symptomatic side. About 50% of patients report the pain along the lateral thigh. Pain is worse with stair climbing and prolonged walking.[11]

8. **Other bursitis**—pain from iliopsoas bursitis is located anteriorly (in the groin) and pain from ischiogluteal bursitis is located posteriorly (buttock) typically; however, diffuse or poorly localized deeply situated pain is also not uncommon.

Iliopsoas bursitis pain is aggravated by the movement involving hip flexion, such as climbing stairs and standing from a sitting position. Snapping with/without pain can occur with hip joint movement.[12] The pain may radiate down to the thigh or to the knee.

Ischiogluteal bursitis can be aggravated by sitting (especially on hard surface) and more common in the person with lean body mass. There is increased friction between the ischial tuberosity and skin in the lean person at sitting because of upward sliding of gluteus maximus muscle surrounding ischiogluteal bursa while sitting.[13]

9. **Stress fracture**—recent increase in activity can raise the suspicion for stress fracture. If there are risk factors, including female athletic triads (irregular menstruation [or amenorrhea], eating disorders, and osteoporosis), or suboptimal biomechanics (leg length discrepancy, coxa vara, etc.), there should be low threshold for imaging study and further workup. Pain is gradual in onset, often located in the groin associated with weight-bearing activity. However, pain can be present at night. Pain is reproduced by extreme range, and hopping (on one leg) and fulcrum test. Often the physical examination is not specific. Once identified, it is important to localize the stress fracture for the management and prognosis. The trabecular pattern of the proximal femur is uniquely arranged to manage forces with medial

trabecular system for vertical compressive forces and lateral trabecular system for shear forces of body weight and ground reaction force (therefore high likelihood of nonunion requiring surgical intervention).

10. **Lumbar spondylosis**—pain from the facet arthropathy from lumbar spondylosis is very common in elderly population. It is located in the midline lower lumbar region, with intermittent referred pain to the buttock and groin. The pain is worse with activity requiring trunk (lumbar) extension and rotation. Flexion of lumbar spine is better tolerated than extension. Neurologic symptoms other than positive sensory symptoms (pain and tingling) are less common; however, they can be seen in the distribution of nerve root that is compromised in the setting of lumbar spondylotic stenosis (with narrowing of neural foramen).

11. **Discogenic pain with radiculopathy**—acute disc herniation at lumbar spine can lead to nerve root compression at this level. Although it is not as common as L5–S1 radiculopathy, it can occur when the lower lumbar spine is less mobile because of degenerative changes or fusion. It is difficult to differentiate the symptoms from L2–L3 radiculopathy versus lumbar radiculoplexus neuropathy (amyotrophy).[14] Lumbar radiculoplexus neuropathy is typically diagnosed as radiculopathy initially and found in 1% of diabetic patients. It involves femoral and sciatic nerves, progresses to the contralateral side , and is associated with weight loss.[14] In both cases, the pain can be severe initially. In radiculoplexus neuropathy, the pain can subside as significant weakness follows.

12. **Malignancy**—if the patient has history of cancer, malignancy (metastatic cancer) should be included as differentials until it is ruled out. It presents with worsening pain at night, in supine position and becomes constant. Systemic manifestation such as weight loss, malaise, fatigue may accompany.[15] When ordering magnetic resonance imaging (MRI), contrast should be added when possible to help further characterize lesions.[16]

13. **Septic arthritis/osteomyelitis**—more common in pediatric population and relatively uncommon in adults (approximate incidence of 4.6 per 100,000).[17] Initially, the presentation can be nonspecific with pain, painful limitation in ROM, and malaise. With risk factors such as drug abuse, hemoglobinopathy, or immunocompromised states, a high index of suspicion is required.[18]

Case Discussion

This patient was an active young adult with insidious onset of hip pain over a few months suggesting chronic nature of conditions. It makes acute traumatic or vascular injury less likely as underlying etiology. Lack of focal neurologic deficit and temporary response to the nonsteroidal antiinflammatory drugs (NSAIDs) suggests musculoskeletal pathologies rather than neurologic disorders. Musculoskeletal pathologies can be divided into the local musculoskeletal pathologies versus distant pathologies causing referred pain to hip (such as lumbar spine, sacroiliac joint complex pathologies, etc.). Among the local pathologies, based on the location of maximal pain and tenderness, the differentials can be further narrowed down (see Table 6.1). Degenerative hip OA is less common in this patient's age group. Considering active lifestyle and sports participation, tendinopathy, strain, sprain, bursitis, chondral, labral, pathology, or other mechanical joint pathology (such as femoroacetabular impingement syndrome) can be considered as the underlying etiology. Intermittent posterior thigh and knee pain indicates either concomitant knee pathology or local hip pathology with referred pain.

It is important to recognize the red flags and order imaging and serologic tests if indicated (e.g., to evaluate inflammatory arthropathies, connective tissue disorders, infections, or tumor/cancer). If there is a reasonable suspicion, then further imaging may be required when the initial imaging findings did not reveal anything.

Objective Data

From the primary care doctor

Complete blood count (CBC)—white blood cell (WBC): 6000 cell/mL; hemoglobin: 12.4 g/dL; within normal limits

Complete metabolic panel—within normal limits

Coagulation panel—within normal limits

Routine x-ray of hip (anteroposterior [AP] pelvis and frog-leg lateral view)—unremarkable. No gross joint space narrowing or osteophyte noted. No gross lucency or sclerosis noted. Sacroiliac joint patent without fusion or sclerosis.

Routine x-ray of spine—degenerative disc disease at L4–5 and L5–S1 levels. Degenerative changes in the lower lumbar facet joints.

Case Discussion

The aforementioned laboratory and imaging data are useful to further narrow down the differential diagnosis. Because the imaging study did not reveal significant findings suggestive of OA and blastic/lytic/sclerotic lesions, moderate to severe OA and metastatic lesion (without the history of cancer) were less likely. However, mild OA/bony deformity, periarticular soft tissue pathologies, and some soft tissue tumors (or early-stage lesion) cannot be completely ruled out by plain x-ray.

CBC and metabolic panel were within normal limits, infection process is also less likely without red flags, but erythrocyte sedimentation rate (ESR) and C-reactive protein (CRP) can be added if there is any suspicion. Serology for gonococcus can be added as well if the sexual history warrants it.

MRI of the hip can be considered if the hip joint pathology is strongly suspected and when the plain x-ray was normal because it can detect subtle bony abnormality and periarticular soft tissue (labral, capsule, ligament, cartilage, etc.) abnormalities. Additional plain x-ray views (such as Dunn/modified Dunn view) can be useful in evaluation of mild bony deformity, such as femoroacetabular impingement syndrome. Computed tomography can be useful in the evaluation of fractures and preoperative planning.

Ultrasonography (US) of the hip is increasingly available in the office setting. Focused US evaluation can be time efficient and useful in some pathologies, such as synovitis/joint effusion, enthesopathy, calcific tendinopathy, tendon, and bursal pathologies.

Because spine pathology is widely prevalent, it may coexist with the hip joint pathology. Alternatively, it can be the culprit of the hip pain (referred pain or radiating pain from the lumbar spine or sacroiliac joint). Positive spine x-ray findings of degenerative changes in lower lumbar spine, in this case, increase this possibility. However, lack of significant low back pain, absence of focal neurologic deficit in the clinical examination, and location of degenerative lumbar pathology (lower lumbar spine level [L4–S1] rather than L2–L3) lower the likelihood of lumbar spine pathology as a main cause of the groin pain although it cannot be completely ruled out. Other neurologic etiologies such as lumbar plexopathy, radiculoplexus-neuropathy (amyotrophy), femoral/obturator mononeuropathy, and myopathy are also low in the clinical suspicion.

Otherwise, the initial management can focus on the conservative treatment.

ADDITIONAL OBJECTIVE DATA

Patient asked to have an MRI because he wanted to know the exact lesion during the visit to primary care doctor (PMD), and subsequently the PMD ordered an MRI.

MRI of hip: Mild joint effusion. Osseous deformity at the transition zone between the femoral head and the femoral neck at the anterior superior hip joint. The alpha angle (on axial view) of the longitudinal axis of the femoral neck and a line between the center of femoral head and the head-neck junction was 65 degrees. There was anterior superior labral tear. There is no other bony or soft tissue abnormality.

Review of Anatomy of the Hip Joint, Proposed Pathology, and Pathobiomechanics of Femoroacetabular Impingement

The hip joint is a ball and socket joint composed of femoral head and acetabulum covering two-thirds of femoral head. Congruence of femoral head and acetabulum contributes to the stability of the hip joint. The stability is reinforced by the labrum, which deepens the acetabular fossa and capsuloligamentous structures around the hip joint. Abnormal congruence can be caused by abnormal morphology of the femoral head-neck junction (cam lesion) or acetabular overcoverage (pincer lesion), which can result in femoroacetabular impingement.[19] Femoroacetabular impingement syndrome (FAI) can lead to the painful loss of ROM and early degenerative joint disease. Other possible etiologies for abnormal contact between proximal femur and acetabulum include previous femoral neck fracture, surgical osteotomy for Legg-Calve-Perthes disease, acetabular retroversion, and slipped capital femoral epiphysis.

Understanding the dynamic joint reaction forces is helpful in understanding the underlying mechanisms of the intermittent nature of symptom in early stage of hip joint pathology (including FAI). The majority of our activities involving hip joint are in the dynamic state rather than true static state (quiet standing without any movement). Hip joint reaction force is the result of the body weight (BW; upper body and trunk) moment and hip joint abductor tension, and ranges from one-third of BW during bipedal stance, 2.5 times BW during walking, and up to more than 8 times of BW during some athletic activity (during tumbling, kicking, jumping, and cutting in). This can explain the intermittent joint mediated symptoms with athletic activity in patients with hip joint pathology, such as FAI (particularly with dynamic impingement position).

FAI can be divided into two distinct types based on the underlying pathomechanism. Cam impingement with nonspherical shape of femoral head causes impingement of femoral head-neck into the acetabulum during hip flexion. Pincer impingement is caused by the increased acetabular coverage (deep acetabulum) of the femoral head abutting femoral head-neck junction by acetabular rim (Fig. 6.1). Both types cause the damage to the intraarticular structures (anterosuperior acetabular cartilage lesion [outside-in pattern] in cam-type and labral damage in the acetabular rim [posteroinferior part] in the pincer type).[19] Because the labrum and capsular/ligamentous complex are important dynamic stabilizers, the injury can cause instability in addition to pain and catching.

CLINICAL SIGNS AND SYMPTOMS

Pain from the hip joint is located in the groin most frequently but can be in the buttock or the side. Pain can vary from dull soreness/ache during athletic activities promoting impingement initially (such as crouching) to constant sharp pain regardless of activity later.

The patient with cam-type FAI demonstrates decreased hip abduction compared with the control group. The pain is worse with hip abductor muscle tension, which varies on the shifting body (mass) over the fulcrum of the hip joint, therefore leaning trunk to the painful hip (Trendelenburg gait) can occur to reduce the joint reaction force.

The mechanical symptoms, such as locking, "giving way" can be present.

ROM is typically limited in hip flexion (average flexion slightly over 90 degrees). Hip flexion, adduction, and internal rotation (FADIR) provokes the symptom (anterior impingement test). Pain can be reproduced by resistive straight leg raise test. Posterior (posteroinferior) impingement test can be done with the symptomatic leg hanging from the end of the examination table while the patient is lying on the bed. The deep groin pain is then reproduced by rotating the hip externally, which is positive for posterior impingement test.[20]

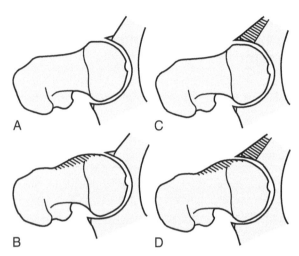

Fig. 6.1 Femoral acetabular impingement types. (A) The normal hip. (B) Cam impingement. (C) Pincer impingement. (D) Combined impingement. (From J.A. Silverstein, J.L. Moeller, M.R. Hutchinson, Common Issues in orthopedics, In: R.E. Rakel, D.P. Rakel (Eds.), Textbook of Family Medicine, 9e, Elsevier, Philadelphia, 2016.)

Groin pain may be referred down to the knee. Negative sensory symptom (numbness) is usually absent. Weakness related to the painful hip joint can be subtle. Weakness related to painful musculoskeletal disorders is typically local with gradual onset and progress. The weakness pattern is quite different from weakness from neuromuscular disorders (involving significant sensory deficit in radiculopathy/plexopathy and contralateral proximal muscles in myopathy). Because both etiologies can coexist, precautions should be applied to delineate the underlying causes.

Deep tendon reflexes are typically normal and symmetric, therefore asymmetric or absent reflexes should raise the suspicion for concomitant neuromuscular pathologies.

IMAGING STUDIES

Plain films are very useful in identifying morphology, deformity, and degenerative hip joint disease. AP view of pelvis and frog-leg lateral view (with hip abduction) are routine views. If there is a trauma, cross-table lateral (because frog-leg lateral view requiring hip abduction is limited because of pain), inlet/outlet view (for pelvic trauma), and Judet view (for acetabular fracture) are indicated.[21,22] In AP view, coccyx should point toward the pubic symphysis within 2 cm (ideally 1 cm) distance to adequately evaluate the acetabulum (true AP view, Fig. 6.2).

For femoroacetabular impingement, Dunn or modified Dunn views (with hip flexed 45 degrees [Dunn] vs. 90 degrees [modified Dunn] and abducted 20 degrees) are used to evaluate the femoral head sphericity or femoral neck anteversion. In this view, acetabular retroversion can show with increased center edge angle (CEA, normal = 25–39 degrees, defined by vertical line drawn through the center of the femoral head and a line drawn from the anterior edge of acetabulum to the center of femoral head) and crossover sign (crossover of anterior and posterior rim; posterior wall medial to the femoral head center [FHC])[23] (Fig. 6.3). Pistol grip deformity and flattened head-neck junction can be seen with cam-type impingement (Fig. 6.4).

In-office musculoskeletal US can be done at bedside to evaluate tendon, muscle injuries, evaluation of effusion/synovitis, and bursal pathologies. It is particularly useful in the enthesopathy and calcific tendinopathy and dynamic evaluation of snapping hip syndrome. However, evaluation of intraarticular structures (labrum and cartilage on femoral head) and subchondral pathology is limited.

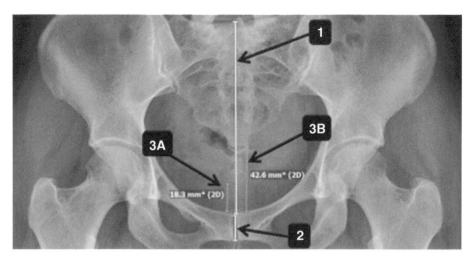

Fig. 6.2 Anteroposterior pelvic radiograph. Lateral rotation can be assessed by *(1)* drawing a line bisecting the sacrum and *(2)* a line bisecting the pubic symphysis. Distance between lines (1) and (2) should be less than 2 cm (ideally 1.0 cm). Pelvic tilt can be assessed by the distance between the superior margin of the pubic symphysis and the tip of the coccyx *(3A)* (normally 1–3 cm) or sacrococcygeal joint *(3B)* (normally 3–5 cm). (From A. Ghaffari, I. Davis, T. Storey, et al., Current concepts of femoroacetabular impingement, Radiol. Clin. North Am. 56 (6) (2018) 965–982, Fig 4.)

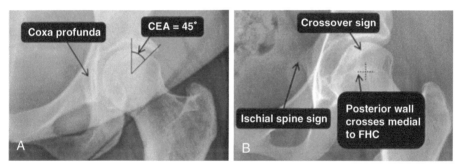

Fig. 6.3 Pincer impingement. (A) Increased center-edge angle *(CEA)* and coxa profunda (the medial border of acetabular fossa medial to the ilioischial line). (B) Crossover sign and ischial spine sign (prominent ischial spine, not obscured by medial acetabulum [normal finding]). Posterior acetabular wall crosses medial to femoral head center *(FHC)*. (From A. Ghaffari, I. Davis, T. Storey, et al., Current concepts of femoroacetabular impingement, Radiol. Clin. North Am. 56 (6) (2018) 965–982, Fig. 11A and B.)

MRI is the gold standard imaging modality for musculoskeletal pathologies, although not always initially indicated. Noncontrast MRI is limited in the evaluation of labral tear, therefore MR arthrogram may be indicated for labral tear and cartilage pathology.[24] MRI can be particularly useful in the subtle bony pathologies, such as subcortical bony edema that can be only signs of early inflammatory arthropathy.[7] In FAI, the alpha angle is frequently measured for cam impingement lesion to determine the contour of the femoral head-neck junction. It is the angle between a line of the center of the femoral head through the middle of the femoral neck and a line from the center of femoral head to the femoral head-neck junction on the axial plane. If the alpha angle is 55 degrees or more, then cam impingement is suspected. The challenge is the lack of correlation between the positive imaging findings in MRI and clinical correlation. For example, 10%

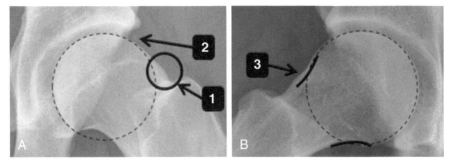

Fig. 6.4 Cam-type morphology on frog-leg lateral radiograph demonstrates cam deformity *(1)* and labral mineralization *(2)*. (B) Asymmetry of the anterior femoral head and neck junction on frog-leg lateral radiograph *(3)*. (From A. Ghaffari, I. Davis, T. Storey, et al., Current concepts of femoroacetabular impingement, Radiol. Clin. North Am. 56 (6) (2018) 965–982, Fig. 12.)

to 25% of young population has the imaging findings suggestive of femoroacetabular impingement (alpha angle ≥55 degrees), however, most of these are asymptomatic.

ELECTROMYOGRAPHY

Patients with painful hip and weakness without clear underlying local (hip) musculoskeletal pathologies can be referred to electromyography (EMG) for evaluation of L2–L3 radiculopathy or lumbar plexopathy (or radiculoplexus-neuropathy). Lack of motor, sensory deficits, and reasonable local musculoskeletal pathologies to explain the patient's symptom, in this case, places EMG unnecessary for initial workup.

DISCUSSION

Morbid conditions, such as infectious, rapidly progressive inflammatory conditions and cancerous etiologies, are unlikely in this case without red flags, suggestive imaging findings, or abnormal serologic test findings although it cannot be completely ruled out, especially in the early stages.

There are no clear clinical indicators for immediate or urgent invasive intervention, such as surgery. Therefore conservative management is strongly advocated as the first line of treatment of FAI. Depending on the level of athletic activities in addition to the patient's symptoms, the treatment decision can be individualized. Because the symptoms are frequently discordant with the radiographic findings, it is important not to be directed by the imaging finding only. An initial management for FAI includes multimodal approach consisting of education, modification of activities, physical therapy, pharmacologic therapy, and injection as needed.

ACUTE PHASE

With worsening of pain, a short period of relative rest from provoking activities (athletic activities or some activities of daily living [ADL]) is beneficial. With significant pain, protected weight bearing using crutch or cane can be tried. Patient is advised to avoid extreme ROM.

Acetaminophen or NSAIDs can be used to alleviate pain temporarily. NSAIDs are known to be more effective than acetaminophen in improving hip pain, function, and global outcome in the patient with hip arthropathy. However, NSAIDs should be used with caution, especially for gastrointestinal adverse effects.[3] Opioid analgesics should be avoided if possible, only reserved for exceptional circumstances (e.g., failed nonpharmacologic intervention, nonopioid analgesics, and not suitable for other local interventions).[25,26] Long-term use should be avoided considering potential serious complications. Three to 6 months of comprehensive multimodal treatment is recommended before surgical evaluation.

Physical Therapy

Physical therapy includes stretching (especially hip flexor), joint mobilization/distraction, strengthening exercise, and neuromuscular training. Stretching should be cautious initially; some considered it counterproductive because it often aggravates the symptom. Progressive strengthening (from isometric initially to gradual resistive strengthening) of gluteal muscles and hip flexor/adductor muscles should be implemented as the flexibility increases. Core muscle stabilization and strengthening exercise are advocated. Coordination and proprioceptive exercise should be emphasized for any joint pathology because joint pathology causes the detrimental effect on the overall balance and joint stability. Also it is important to emphasize that one of the principles of physical therapy is to educate the patient to learn the therapeutic exercise routine and to continue it at home. However, the evidence supporting conservative management of FAI is still weak.[27]

Injection

When the pain is persistent despite the course of education, physical therapy, and oral analgesics, image-guided hip joint injection can be considered for short-term pain relief. Recently, alternatives to steroid injection have been tried, including hyaluronic acid or platelet-rich plasma injection with limited evidence for efficacy. In addition to the therapeutic effect, image-guided injection can confirm the origin of the pain from the hip joint complex (such as labrum) in a patient with challenging diagnosis (such as one with concomitant lumbar pathology).[28] For chronic recalcitrant pain in patients who are poor candidates for surgery, nerve block can be considered as an option to manage pain. The branches from obturator nerve and femoral nerve can be the target for nerve block or ablation therapy, typically done under imaging guidance.

Referral to Surgery

If a patient fails to respond to nonoperative therapy after at least a 6-month period with an inability to maintain ADLs or athletic activities with significant compromise in quality of life, then a referral for surgical intervention is warranted. Surgical options include open or arthroscopic procedure to debride the labrum in painful labral tear, remove some of the femur (osteoplasty), and/or acetabular osteotomy. The possible complications include peripheral nerve injury, trochanteric nonunion, osteonecrosis of the femoral head, and femoral neck fracture. Understanding the recovery process and restricted activities after the surgical procedure can be also useful to plan the treatment from patient's (especially athlete) perspective. Systemic review by Reiman et al. showed one in four athletes did not return to their previous level of sports activities after surgical interventions. So far, there are no clear predictors for surgical outcomes available, therefore predicting the prognosis of return to sports is difficult.[29]

Summary

A patient presents with chronic hip pain, worsening over time without focal neurologic symptoms and signs (weakness, numbness) along with demonstrable clinical signs of FAI. The patient initially had routine x-ray of the hip, which was within normal limits. Further testing (Dunn view) revealed cam type of FAI and MRI of the hip confirmed FAI with labral tear. He stopped athletic activities and pain was managed with NSAIDs without great success. Diagnostic/therapeutic hip joint injection and physical therapy were implemented with good response to the conservative management. At a follow-up visit 3 months later, patient remained pain free and without limitations in ADL. He uses an occasional Tylenol and began gradual return to play protocol.

Key Points

- Hip pain can be from multiple different etiologies requiring careful assessment.
- History and physical examination can delineate the differential diagnosis and can help to create a therapeutic plan of care.
- Treatment options should be tailored to individual patient, including modification of activities, avoidance of provoking activities, therapeutic exercise, injection, and referral to surgery.

CLINICAL PEARLS

The pain from hip osteoarthritis is often vague, most commonly in the groin but can be in the lateral and posterior aspect (buttock pain, up to 71%) possibly with referred leg pain.

Femoroacetabular impingement can be divided into cam impingement with nonspherical shape of femoral head impinging the acetabulum during hip flexion and pincer impingement with increased acetabular coverage of the femoral head abutting femoral head-neck junction by acetabular rim.

Image-guided hip joint injection can be useful for confirming the origin of the pain from the hip joint complex (such as labrum) in a patient with challenging diagnosis.

References

1. E.C. Falvey, A. Franklyn-Miller, P.R. McCrory, The groin triangle: a patho-anatomical approach to the diagnosis of chronic groin pain in athletes, Br. J. Sports Med. 43 (3) (2009) 213–220.
2. P. Suri, D.C. Morgenroth, D.J. Hunter, Epidemiology of osteoarthritis and associated comorbidities, Pharm. Manag. PM R 4 (5, Suppl. ment) (2012) S10–S19.
3. N. Aresti, J. Kassam, N. Nicholas, P. Achan, Hip osteoarthritis, BMJ 354 (2016) i3405.
4. J.M. Leshe, P. Dreyfus, N. Hager, M. Kapan, M. Furman, Hip joint pain referral patterns: a descriptive study, Pain Med. 9 (1) (2008) 22–25.
5. J.W.T. Byrd, Evaluation of the hip: history and physical examination, North Am. J. Sports Phys. Ther. 2 (4) (2007) 231–240.
6. W.N. Sankar, T.H. Matheney, I. Zaltz, Femoroacetabular impingement: current concepts and controversies, Orthop. Clin. North Am. 44 (4) (2013) 575–589.
7. C. Schueller-Weidekamm, J. Teh, Inflammatory conditions of the hip, Semin. Musculoskelet. Radiol. 21 (5) (2017) 589–603.
8. A. Cianci, D. Sugimoto, A. Stracciolini, Y.M. Yen, M.S. Kocher, P.A. d'Hemecourt, Nonoperative management of labral tears of the hip in adolescent athletes: description of sports participation, interventions, comorbidity, and outcomes, Clin. J. Sport. Med. 29 (1) (2019) 24–28.
9. S.J. Parsons, N. Steele, Osteonecrosis of the femoral head: Part 1—Aetiology, pathogenesis, investigation, classification, Curr. Orthop. 21 (6) (2007) 457–463.
10. D. Resnick, G. Niwayama, Diagnosis of Bone and Joint Disorders, vols. 1–6, 1988.
11. B. Rothschild, Trochanteric area pain, the result of a quartet of bursal inflammation, World J. Orthop. 4 (3) (2013) 100–102.
12. C.N. Anderson, Iliopsoas: pathology, diagnosis, and treatment, Clin. Sports Med. 35 (3) (2016) 419–433.
13. I.M. Van Mieghem, A. Boets, R. Sciot, I. van Breuseghem, Ischiogluteal bursitis: an uncommon type of bursitis, Skeletal Radiol. 33 (7) (2004) 413–416.
14. E.P. McCormack, M. Alam, N.J. Erickson, A.A. Cherrick, E. Powell, J.H. Sherman, Use of MRI in diabetic lumbosacral radiculoplexus neuropathy: case report and review of the literature, Acta. Neurochir. (Wien) 160 (11) (2018) 2225–2227.
15. J.L. Bloem, I.I. Reidsma, Bone and soft tissue tumors of hip and pelvis, Eur. J. Radiol. 81 (12) (2012) 3793–3801.
16. D. Nascimento, G. Suchard, M. Hatem, A. de Abreu, The role of magnetic resonance imaging in the evaluation of bone tumours and tumour-like lesions, Insights Imaging 5 (4) (2014) 419–440.

17. Y.K. Lee, K.S. Park, Y.C. Ha, K.H. Koo, Arthroscopic treatment for acute septic arthritis of the hip joint in adults, Knee Surg. Sports Traumatol. Arthrosc. 22 (4) (2014) 942–945.
18. L. Nallamshetty, J.M. Buchowski, L.A. Nazarian, et al., Septic arthritis of the hip following cortisone injection: case report and review of the literature, Clin. Imaging 27 (4) (2003) 225–228.
19. R. Sutter, C.W.A. Pfirrmann, Update on femoroacetabular impingement: what is new, and how should we assess it? Semin. Musculoskelet. Radiol. 21 (5) (2017) 518–528.
20. J. Parvizi, M. Leunig, R. Ganz, Femoroacetabular impingement, J. Am. Acad. Orthop. Surg. 15 (9) (2007) 561–570.
21. J.C. Clohisy, J.C. Carlisle, P.E. Beaulé, et al., A systematic approach to the plain radiographic evaluation of the young adult hip, J. Bone Joint Surg. 90 (Suppl. 4) (2008) 47–66.
22. S.-J. Lim, Y.-S. Park, Plain radiography of the hip: a review of radiographic techniques and image features, Hip Pelvis 27 (3) (2015) 125–134.
23. A. Ghaffari, I. Davis, T. Storey, M. Moser, Current concepts of femoroacetabular impingement, Radiol. Clin. North Am. 56 (6) (2018) 965–982.
24. T.T. Miller, Abnormalities in and around the hip: MR imaging versus sonography, Magn. Reson. Imaging. Clin. N. Am. 13 (4) (2005) 799–809.
25. D.J. Hunter, S. Bierma-Zeinstra, Osteoarthritis. Lancet 393 (10182) (2019) 1745–1759.
26. C. Zeng, M. Dubreuil, M.R. LaRochelle, et al., Association of tramadol with all-cause mortality among patients with osteoarthritis, J. Am. Med. Assoc. 321 (10) (2019) 969–982.
27. P.D. Wall, M. Fernandez, D.R. Griffin, N.E. Foster, Nonoperative treatment for femoroacetabular impingement: a systematic review of the literature, Pharm. Manag. PMR 5 (5) (2013) 418–426.
28. O.R. Ayeni, F. Farrokhyar, S. Crouch, K. Chan, S. Sprague, M. Bhandari, Pre-operative intra-articular hip injection as a predictor of short-term outcome following arthroscopic management of femoroacetabular impingement, Knee Surg. Sports Traumatol. Arthrosc. 22 (4) (2014) 801–805.
29. M.P. Reiman, S. Peters, J. Sylvain, S. Hagymasi, R.C. Mather, A.P. Goode, Femoroacetabular impingement surgery allows 74% of athletes to return to the same competitive level of sports participation but their level of performance remains unreported: a systematic review with meta-analysis, Br. J. Sports Med. 52 (15) (2018) 972–981.
30. K.M. de Bruijn, G. Franssen, T.M. van Ginhoven, A stepwise approach to 'groin pain': a common symptom, an uncommon cause, BMJ Case Rep. 2013 (2013).

CHAPTER 7

Elbow Pain

Dr. Subhadra Nori, MD ▪ Dr. Jasmine H. Harris, MD

Case Presentation

A 58-year-old, right-hand dominant male is referred to the Physical Medicine and Rehabilitation (PM&R) clinic from his primary care provider for right elbow pain. His pain is located on the medial aspect of his elbow. The pain started 4 months ago and was a dull and achy sensation initially but has worsened to a sharp pain radiating to his inner forearm for 1 month. He notes pain is 6 on a 10-point visual analogue scale. He has occasional numbness and tingling in the medial aspect of his palm and pinky finger for the past 3 weeks which was not present in preceding months. Pain at times wakes him up from his sleep. He does not recall any inciting event, trauma, or accidents. He denies any neck pain, arm, or hand weakness. He has taken ibuprofen which helped initially but now provides minimal pain relief.

REVIEW OF SYSTEMS

Past medical history: He has a history of diabetes for which he is on metformin 500 mg daily for the past 15 years and knee osteoarthritis

Social history: He works as a mechanic. He is widowed and lives in a private house with his 22-year-old son. He smokes 3 to 4 cigarettes per day.

Past surgical history: Tonsillectomy at 13 years of age

Allergies: Shellfish, pollen

Medications: Metformin 500 mg bid, occasional Tylenol and ibuprofen

Vitals: BP: 128/78 mmHg, HR: 72 beats per min, RR: 14/min, Temp: 98.2° F, Ht: 5'10", Wt: 235 lbs, BMI 32.2 kg/m^2

Examination

General: Obese middle aged man, appears in mild distress, alert

Head, eyes, ear, nose, and throat (HEENT)-PERRLA-extraocular movements (EOM) intact, no ptosis, anicteric sclera

Extremities: No edema, no skin rashes, no surgical scars, no fasciculations seen on C spine

Full range of motion (ROM) of C-spine in all directions

Manual muscle testing: 5/5 shoulder abduction, elbow flexion and extension, wrist extension, finger abduction, finger flexion but giveway because of pain with resisted wrist flexion and pronation on the right fist grip intact bilaterally

Deep tendon reflexes 1+ Biceps, BR, triceps bilaterally, negative Hoffman

Tone normal

2+ radial pulses

Sensation: Intact to light touch in arm and forearm in all dermatomes, diminished light touch over dorsal and palmar ulnar aspect of the little and ring finger

Musculoskeletal pain with palpation at the medial epicondyle

No muscle atrophy, no deformities

Full ROM of elbow but pain at end of range of elbow flexion, shoulder, and wrist

Gait normal, nonantalgic

Laboratories: White blood cell (WBC) 6.5 H/H 34/13, blood urea nitrogen (BUN)/creatinine (Cr) 21/0.9, hemoglobin (Hgb)A1c 6.4%

General Discussion

There are several causes of medial elbow pain. A differential diagnosis should be generated as an initial approach to identify the most likely condition(s). One should be aware of the potential for more than one condition present at the same time. Medical history should include questions about recent trauma, surgery, illness, and intravenous (IV) drug use. Physical examination should include examination of cervical spine, shoulder, elbow, wrist, and hand with comparison to the unaffected side. Report of numbness and/or tingling of the hands and an abnormal sensory examination should prompt further investigation for possible nerve compression.

Differential Diagnosis

Medial epicondylitis (ME)—also known as golfer's elbow. Patient complains of pain over the medial epicondyle. Caused by repetitive valgus stress, flexion leading to inflammation of the common flexor tendon, and hypertrophy of medial epicondyle. Pain is reproduced with flexion and pronation. May involve an associated ulnar nerve neuropathy[1] (Fig. 7.1).

Ulnar collateral ligament (UCL) sprain—typically seen with overhead athletes, such as baseball pitchers, tennis players, football quarterbacks, and volleyball players. It is also important not to overlook an associated UCL tear.

Cubital tunnel syndrome—common medial elbow pain found in athletes and manual laborers or workers exposed to repetitive motion. The incidence is quite high and is reported at a rate of 0.8% per person-year in laborers.[4] Cubital tunnel is formed by the medial epicondyle medially, olecranon process posteriorly, and bordered by the Osborne ligament and the ulnar collateral ligaments. The ulnar nerve passes through this tunnel and is vulnerable for compression.

Osteochondritis dissecans (OCD)—is defined as an inflammatory condition of bone and cartilage. This can result in localized necrosis and fragmentation of bone and cartilage. OCD of the elbow is most commonly seen in the adolescent population (ages 12-14) in particular throwing sports or upper limb dominant sports such as baseball or hockey; hence the common term little leaguer elbow.[16]

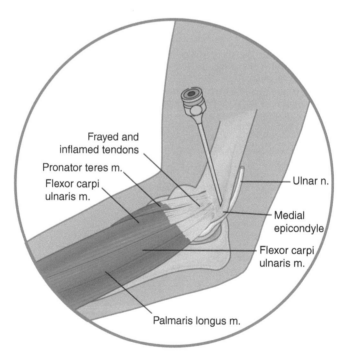

Fig. 7.1 Medial elbow anatomic structures. (S.D. Waldman, Atlas of Pain Management Injection Techniques, 3e, Elsevier, Philadelphia, 2012, Fig. 49-3.)

In the elbow, the most common area affected is the capitellum, although it has been reported to affect the olecranon and the trochlea. One or more flakes of articular cartilage have become separated. These form loose bodies within the joint. The separated flakes can then ossify due to nourishment by the synovial fluid. The cartilage is damaged and can form a loose body. Conservative management, analgesia, NSAIDs, and bracing to offload the joint are indicated. Treatment includes a hinged brace set to a pain-free range of movement (ROM), ceasing sports or activities that aggravate symptoms for 6-12 weeks, activity modification, and occupational therapy (OT).[17]

Surgical management: Arthroscopic surgery will aim to assess the anterior elbow, remove loose bodies and fragments, debride any necrotic bone to stimulate increased blood flow. A large fragment may need to be reattached to the capitellum via K wire or screw fixation. In severe cases, osteochondral grafting may be required.[18,19]

Ulnohumeral osteoarthritis —presents as pain in the elbow. Affects women >men in early osteoarthritis, patients complain of elbow pain at the extremes of flexion and extension. At maximum extension, degenerative osteophytes on the olecranon impinge with osteophytes present on the olecranon fossa. At maximum flexion, osteophytes of the trochlea and coronoid cause impingement. Coupled with pain, elbow stiffness and ROM are due to these impinging osteophytes and the capsular contracture that commonly develops during the disease process. Mechanical symptoms such as catching and locking may be present due to the presence of intraarticular loose bodies. In addition to pain with ROM, patients with elbow arthritis often report an inability to carry heavy objects.

Treatment is pain relief with NSAIDs, physical/occupational therapy for modalities, ROM exercises, bracing and position modifying techniques, elbow bracing for unloading. If conservative management fails, surgical ulnohumeral arthroplasty, open osteocapsular debridement, and/or arthroscopic debridement are recommended for patients with impingement symptoms and pain at the extremes of motion and those with mild to moderate degenerative changes associated with restricted ROM short of the functional range. For patients older than 60-65 years, total elbow arthroplasty is considered the treatment of choice, and for those who complain of a painful elbow with a restricted ROM in the setting of significant degenerative changes

Occult fracture —can occur because of a fall or other type of sudden (acute) injury. Such fractures can also occur because of repetitive injuries or normal stresses on weak bones such as osteoporotic bones, Fractures caused by repetitive injuries are fatigue fractures. Those that result from normal stresses on weak bones are insufficiency fractures. Another name for these fractures is stress fractures. These features can be induced by long-term steroid use. MRI is one of the best tools for diagnosing occult fractures. Treatment depends on the cause. Bracing is helpful. If conservative management fails patient may need surgical fixation.

Case Discussion

The patient reports no preceding trauma or illness. Cervical spine should be evaluated to rule out other causes of neuropathy. The intrinsic muscles of the hand should be examined for muscle atrophy as may be seen with ulnar nerve pathology. The active and passive ROM of the elbow may be used as a dynamic evaluation of any abnormalities that may contribute to nerve compression. Two-point discrimination involves the use of monofilaments to accurately test the loss of a patient's sensation. Motor strength in all upper extremity muscle groups is tested, with particular focus on grip strength and the ability to abduct fingers against resistance. Provocative tests include the Tinel sign, which is positive if the patient experiences a tingling sensation in the ulnar nerve distribution when the ulnar nerve is percussed proximally at the elbow. Elbow flexion-compression test is another provocative

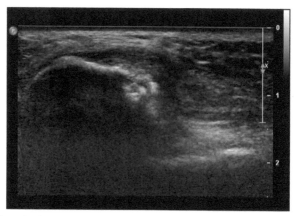

Fig. 7.2 Calcifications in the common flexor tendon. (From A.M. Highland, Imaging of the elbow, In: D. Stanley, I. Trail (Eds.), Operative Elbow Surgery, Elsevier, Philadelphia, 2012, 67–89, Fig. 5-7.)

test, which is positive if the patient experiences numbness in the ulnar nerve distribution while the elbow is flexed. Other tests include the compression test and ulnar nerve subluxation.

ME is typically seen in 40- to 60-year-olds. Besides athletes, it is a common occupational disorder with a prevalence as high as 5%. There is a common association between ME and ulnar neuropathy at the elbow with a range in prevalence from 23% to 61%.[2] Classification of ME is related to the presence and severity of concomitant ulnar neuropathy. Type 1 includes epitroch-leitis without neuropathy, type IIA includes symptomatic patients without deficit, and type IIB include patients with clinical deficit and electromyographic changes.[3]

Cubital tunnel syndrome is common medial elbow pain found in athletes and manual labor-ers or workers exposed to repetitive motion. The incidence of cubital tunnel syndrome is quite high and is reported at a rate of 0.8% per person year in laborers[4] (Fig. 7.2). Paresthesia of the ulnar hand can also result from C8/T1 radicular compression, lower trunk or medial cord brachial plexopathy, thoracic outlet syndrome, or ulnar nerve compression within the Guyon canal at the wrist or at the cubital tunnel at the elbow.[5] Patients who have cervical radiculopathy generally report neck pain radiating into the arm, sensory changes, and weakness in ulnar and median innervated muscles, such as the thumb abductors (median innervated) and finger extensors (radial innervated), with sensory changes that extend into the medial forearm.

Objective Data

CB—within normal limits
Coagulation panel—within normal limits
Complete metabolic panel—within normal limits

ELECTROMYOGRAPHY

Nerve conduction study reveals normal median and ulnar sensory and motor responses, including latencies, amplitudes, and nerve conduction velocities at the wrist. However, there is a decrease in conduction velocity to 38 m/s of the ulnar response across the elbow. There was no significant difference in sensory latencies among the median and radial responses. Needle electromyography (EMG) reveals no abnormal spontaneous activity in the abductor pollicis brevis (APB), abductor digiti minimi (ADM), or cervical paraspinal muscles. These findings suggest an ulnar neuropathy.

Review of Proposed Pathology and Pathobiomechanics

The elbow is a synovial hinge joint formed by the articulation between the olecranon of the ulna and the trochlea of the humerus. The elbow is stabilized by the joint capsule, ulnar collateral ligaments, and the flexor and extensor muscles of the forearm. Injury to any one of these structures leads to increased stress on the others. The muscles of the flexor-pronator group include the pronator teres, flexor carpi radialis, palmaris longus, flexor digitorum superficialis, and flexor carpi ulnaris. The flexor carpi radialis, palmaris longus, and flexor carpi ulnaris form the common flexor tendon (CFT).[2] ME involves degenerative changes at the common flexor tendon, but more specifically involves the pronator teres and the flexor carpi radialis. The pronator teres humeral head origin off the medial conjoined tendon has been implicated as the focal point for the development of ME.[4] The pathologic features of ME are similar to those of lateral epicondylitis and include degeneration, angiofibroblastic change, and an inadequate reparative response, leading to tendinosis and tearing.

The risk factors associated with occupation and ME included handling loads more than 5 kg at least for 2 hours per day or loads more than 20 kg at least 10 times per day, high hand grip forces for more than 1 hour per day, repetitive movements for more than 2 hours per day, and using vibrating tools for more than 2 hours per day.[5]

ME is classified into two major subtypes: type 1 with no ulnar involvement and type 2 with ulnar nerve involvement. The prognosis for type 2 ME is worse than the prognosis for type 1 and it is for this reason that careful diagnosis and treatment of patients with ulnar nerve symptoms frequently determine outcome.

On the dorsomedial elbow, the ulnar nerve travels in the cubital tunnel which is a space located between the medial epicondyle of the humerus, olecranon process of the ulna, Osborne ligament, and medial collateral ligaments (MCLs).[6] Cubital tunnel syndrome may be found with occupations that involve constant holding of a tool in a position and performing repetitive movements.[7] Patients who are obese and have diabetes are also at increased risk. Diabetes leads to a microvascular nerve injury leading to altered metabolism local ischemia or by interfering with the innate metabolism of the nerve.[8]

Clinical Signs and Symptoms of Epicondylitis and Mononeuropathy

Symptoms of ME are described as intermittent pain localized around the medial epicondyle usually associated with activity. Episodes occur for more than 4 of 7 days. On examination, pain is reproduced with wrist flexion or pronation, and/or valgus stress. Patients may complain of night pain and pain at rest. Associated cubital tunnel syndrome will be described with intermittent paresthesia in the fourth and fifth digit or ulnar aspect of the forearm, wrist, and hand. Paresthesia may be reproduced with resistance of the forearm, wrist, or hand and a positive combined pressure and flexion test. Testing of the cubital tunnel involves elbow flexion and direct pressure on the ulnar nerve. It is important to evaluate for any sensory loss in the ulnar digits or intrinsic weakness in more severe cases.

ELECTROMYOGRAPHY

EMG can help to localize the site of entrapment and exclude other diagnoses, such as cervical radiculopathy or brachial plexopathy. Ulnar neuropathy at the elbow is suggestive with slow conduction velocity across the elbow on motor nerve conduction studies, indicating a conduction block with focal demyelination. Sensory, mixed ulnar nerve conduction studies, and segmental stimulation studies may be used to localize the lesion. Needle EMG may also help in localizing the lesion.[9] If there is severe nerve damage, spontaneous activity with fibrillation potentials and positive sharp waves can be seen in muscles innervated by the ulnar nerve followed by severely diminished motor units in the affected muscles.

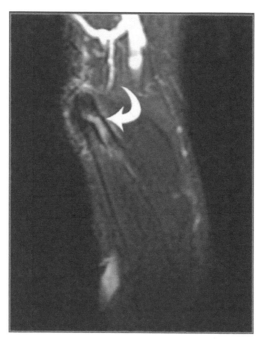

Fig. 7.3 US imaging of the medial elbow. *(Curved arrow)* Increased signal intensity with surrounding fluid in the medial epicondyle/CFT area. (From G. Abrams, M. Safran, Presentation, Imaging and Treatment of Common Musculoskeletal Conditions, Saunders, Philadelphia, 2011, 133–135, Fig. 32-2.)

IMAGING STUDIES

Imaging may not be essential in the initial evaluation of ME. In cases of refractory symptoms unresponsive to conservative management or if there is suspicion for confounding pathologies, imaging would be recommended. Radiographs may appear normal but may show calcification adjacent to the medial epicondyle are useful for evidence of bony impingement, osteoarthritis, and prior trauma.[10]

Magnetic resonance imaging (MRI) and ultrasound may also be used. MRI is preferred if there are signs of ulnar nerve involvement. Ulnar neuritis is identified as thickening and increased signal intensity of the nerve on T2-weighted images.[2] MRI may also be helpful in identifying other soft tissue abnormalities, such as masses, thickened retinaculum, as well as abnormalities of the flexor-pronator mass, intraarticular loose bodies, MCL injury, and ulnar nerve entrapment. Tendon thickening with increased signal intensity indicates tendinosis. Also consider imaging the brachial plexus and cervical spine to exclude other diagnoses.

Ultrasonography (US) helps to evaluate pathologic conditions of the elbow. Musculoskeletal US is a noninvasive dynamic imaging technique that can also be used to image the ulnar nerve.[11] Ultrasound can identify effusions, loose bodies, full or partial thickness tears. At sonography tendinosis appears as hypoechogenicity and possible tendon enlargement (>4.2 mm for lateral extensor tendon). Calcifications and bony irregularities are also seen. Hyperemia on color or power Doppler from neovascularity correlates with patient symptoms[12] (Fig. 7.3).

MRI provides clinically useful information in assessing the elbow joint. Superior depiction of muscles, ligaments, and tendons, as well as the ability to directly visualize nerves, bone marrow, and hyaline cartilage are advantages of MRI relative to conventional imaging techniques. Ongoing improvements in surface coil design and newer pulse sequences have resulted in higher quality

MRI of the elbow. Traumatic and degenerative disorders of the elbow are well seen with MRI. The sequelae of medial traction and lateral compression from valgus stress include MCL injury, common flexor tendon pathology, medial traction spurs, ulnar neuropathy, and osteochondritis dissecans.

Discussion

ACUTE PHASE

Treatment of cubital tunnel syndrome is generally conservative for at least 6 months. In addition, 90% of patients will have resolution of symptoms with conservative management of epicondylitis. Conservative management includes rest, ice, nonsteroidal antiinflammatory drugs (NSAIDs), and physical therapy.[13]

Initially resting from any provoking activity is necessary. Complete immobilization is avoided as to avoid disuse atrophy. Applying ice for 20 minutes three to four times a day is recommended for local vasoconstrictive and analgesic effects.[14]

Other treatment options for ME are acupuncture, orthotic devices, laser therapy, electrotherapy, exercises, and mobilization techniques, but the effectiveness of these therapies is unknown.

PHARMACOTHERAPY

Oral NSAIDs may be prescribed for pain relief and may be administered for 1 to 2 weeks if there are no medical contraindications and if patient is able to tolerate. The beneficial effects of antiinflammatory medications are thought to result from its effect in relieving pain associated with accompanying peritendinous synovitis. Night splinting should emphasize splinting the elbow in extension for patients with ulnar neuritis.[14]

PHYSICAL THERAPY AND MANIPULATION

Physical therapy is essential in recovery. Rehabilitative stretching and strengthening exercises are progressively implemented. A full, painless ROM in the wrist and elbow is initiated. Passive ROM and eccentric contraction are avoided initially to prevent applying unintended excessive stress on the tendon. Once a painless functional motion arc is achieved, tendon strengthening begins. Concentric open and closed chain exercises are used, with increasing weight and repetitions to increase flexor-pronator mass power. Finally, eccentric strengthening of the elbow flexors is implemented.[15]

STEROID INJECTIONS

Steroids have been used in the treatment of epicondylitis, but the literature supporting their efficacy is inconclusive. Corticosteroid injections are effective for short-term (6 weeks or less) pain relief, increase of grip strength, and overall improvement, but do not provide intermediate or long-term effects. In chronic epicondylitis, platelet-rich plasma (PRP) has been shown to effectively reduce pain and symptoms.[16]

Chronic Phase

REFERRAL TO SURGERY

If conservative therapies are unsuccessful, one should consider surgical management. Depending on the severity of symptoms, different surgical options are available. For mild symptoms of ME, a medial epicondylectomy provides significant symptom relief. The simultaneous release of the common flexor origin with decompression of the ulnar nerve helps to improve long-term ulnar nerve function.[4]

Summary

A patient presented with chronic elbow pain, particularly in the medial elbow. He demonstrated symptoms and signs suggestive of medial common flexor tendon dysfunction. Further evaluation included x-ray and ultrasound imaging which confirmed the diagnosis. Initially, he received occupational therapy consisting of stretching, and an US to the medial epicondyle. He was begun on an intrinsic muscle strengthening program, was educated on wearing the orthotic, and starting a home exercise program focusing on flexor muscle stretching. At 4 weeks follow-up, he reported only mild improvement and was then referred for US-guided injection to the medial epicondyle with 1 cc of Depo-Medrol and 2 cc of lidocaine, to which he improved significantly. He still uses the forearm brace and uses modifications in his grip style. Muscle strength has improved slightly.

Key Points

- Underlying etiologies of elbow pain are diverse and classified into musculoskeletal versus neuropathic and regional versus distant pain generators. The structural approach is useful to differentiate complex etiologies.
- Careful attention should be placed to all elements of the history and examination, including the location of the pain, tenderness, evaluation of biomechanics, provocating tests, and functional tests.
- Treatment options should be tailored to individual patients, including education, bracing, therapeutic exercise, precise injections, or surgical referral, and special consideration given to the activity level of the individual and whether return to work or sports is involved.

References

1. S. Di Giacomo, et al., Management of epicondylitis and epitrochleitis, In: G. Porcellini, R. Rotini, S. Stignani Kantar, S. Di Giacomo (Eds.), The Elbow, Springer, Cham, 2018.
2. D.M. Walz, J.S. Newman, G.P. Konin, G. Ross, Epicondylitis: pathogenesis, imaging, and treatment, Radiographics 30 (1) (2010) 167–184.
3. R.M. van Rijn, B.M.A. Huisstede, B.W. Koes, A. Burdorf, Associations between work-related factors and specific disorders at the elbow: a systematic literature review, Rheumatol. 48 (5) (2009) 528–536.
4. C. Brady, A. Dutta, Medial epicondylitis and medial elbow pain syndrome: current treatment strategies, J. Musculoskelet. Disord. Treat 2 (2016) 014.
5. R.M. van Rijn, B.M.A. Huisstede, B.W. Koes, A. Burdorf, Associations between work-related factors and specific disorders at the elbow: a systematic literature review, Rheumatology 48 (5) (2009) 528–536.
6. K. Eberlin, Y. Marjoua, J. Jupiter, Compressive neuropathy of the ulnar nerve: a perspective on history and current controversies, J. Hand Surg. Am. 42 (6) (2017) 464–469.
7. A. Descatha, A. Leclerc, J.F. Chastang, et al., Incidence of ulnar nerve entrapment at the elbow in repetitive work, Scand. J. Work. Environ. Health 30 (2004) 234–240.
8. S. Cutts, Cubital tunnel syndrome, Postgrad. Med. J. 83 (975) (2007) 28–31.
9. B.E. Shapiro, D.C. Preston, Entrapment and compressive neuropathies, Med. Clin. North Am. 93 (2) (2009) 285–315.
10. S. Blease, D.W. Stoller, M.R. Safran, A.E Li, R.C. Fritz, The elbow, In: D.W. Stoller, ed., Magnetic resonance imaging in orthopaedics and sports medicine. 3e. Lippincott, Williams & Wilkins, Philadelphia, 2007, 1463–1626.
11. G.P. Konin, L.N. Nazarian, D.M. Walz, US of the elbow: indications, technique, normal anatomy and pathologic conditions, Radiographics 33 (4) (2013) E125–E147.
12. J.A. Jacobson, Fundamentals of Musculoskeletal Ultrasound, 3e, Elsevier, Philadelphia, 2018.
13. S.F. Kane, J.H. Lynch, J.C. Taylor, Evaluation of elbow pain in adults, Am. Fam. Physician 89 (8) (2014) 649–657.

14. M.G. Ciccotti, M.N. Ramani, Medial epicondylitis, Tech. Hand Up. Extrem. Surg. 7 (4) (2003) 190–196.
15. N.H. Amin, et al., Medial epicondylitis: evaluation and management, J. Am. Acad. Orthopaed. Surg. 23 (6) (2015) 348.
16. M.C. Ciccotti, M.A. Schwartz, M.G. Ciccotti, Diagnosis and treatment of medial epicondylitis of the elbow. Clin. Sports Med. 23 (2004), 693–705.

CHAPTER 8

Foot and Ankle Pain

Dr. Se Won Lee, MD ▪ Dr. Mohammed Emam, MD

Case Presentation

A 57-year-old African-American woman presents to the Physical Medicine and Rehabilitation (PM&R) clinic complaining of right-sided foot and ankle pain with no preceding injury or trauma. The pain has been present for about 9 months and is gradually worsening. She reports that her pain is constant, aggravated by prolonged standing and walking. She takes occasional naproxen which seems to help temporarily. There is mild swelling in the right ankle. She denies any pins/needles sensation or numbness. Her daily activities, including walking and her job duties, are interrupted because of the pain. She denies any focal weakness in the lower extremities. Her review of systems is significant for intermittent low back pain, otherwise negative. She was seen by her primary care doctor and had x-ray imaging of the foot and ankle.

Past medical history: She has a history of hypertension (HTN) for which she is on hydrochlorothiazide, 25 mg O.D. for the past 10 years. She is postmenopausal.

Past surgical history: Lumbar spine surgery (decompression and fusion) 4 years ago.

Social history: She works as a sales manager, lives with her family (husband and one daughter) in an elevator accessible apartment on the fourth floor.

Allergies: No known drug allergy.

Medications: Hydrochlorothiazide, 25 mg O.D., occasional Naproxen.

BP: 130/72 mmHg, RR: 18/min, PR: 72 per min, Temp: 97.4° F, Ht: 5'6", Wt: 180 lbs, BMI 29 kg/m^2

PHYSICAL EXAMINATION

General: She is alert and oriented to person, place, and time. A well-developed, obese lady without significant distress.

Extremities: No skin rashes, surgical scars, or open wounds. Bilateral genu valgum. Bilateral pes planus.

MUSCULOSKELETAL EXAMINATION

Range of motion (ROM) of the lumbar spine: Within functional limits, however, mild pain is reported in the midline of the lower lumbar spine with extension.

Motor exam: 5/5 and symmetric in all muscles groups of bilateral upper and lower extremities.

Deep tendon reflexes (DTR) exam: 2+ in both upper and lower extremities.

Sensory exam: Intact to light touch and pinprick in all dermatomes in both lower extremities.

Gait: No gross foot-dragging or slapping.

Straight leg raise test: Negative.

Patrick (flexion, abduction, and external rotation) test: Negative.

Ely test: Tight rectus femoris on the right side.

No tenderness at the greater trochanters bilaterally

ROM of the knee: Within functional limits.

ROM of the ankle with subtalar neutral: Within functional limits except for heel cord tightness on ankle dorsiflexion.

Foot and ankle palpation: tenderness at the medial hindfoot between the medial malleolus and navicular tuberosity

Silfverskiold test: Positive (more than 10-degree change of ankle dorsiflexion on knee flexion from knee extension [with limited ankle dorsiflexion <5 degrees])[1] on both sides.

Double heel-rise test: Intact.

Single heel-rise test: Impaired hindfoot (heel) inversion on the right side and intact on the left side.

Labs: White blood cell (WBC): 6000 cell/mL; hemoglobin (Hg): 12.6 g/dL

The General Approach to Foot and Ankle Pain

During the approach to a patient with gradual onset of foot and ankle pain, the initial focus should be to differentiate local pathologies from pain referred from proximal pain generators, such as lumbar, hip, or knee pathologies. It is also important to differentiate between musculoskeletal and neuropathic pain generators.

If proximal pain generators, such as the spine, hip, and knee pathologies are ruled out, then local foot and ankle pathologies can be further classified based on the location of maximal pain and tenderness.

Frequently, patients can present with multiple independent pathologies in different parts of the lower extremities that can be caused by similar faulty biomechanics. Taking into consideration the closed kinetic chain during functional activities (such as standing and walking), recognizing faulty biomechanics is important for diagnosis, understanding underlying etiologies, and planning the treatment.

It is also important to recognize if there are any red flags that would prompt urgent imaging and further investigation.

The physical examination can follow the aforementioned sequences by localizing the pain generators in the foot and ankle region. Tenderness can be a compass to the local pain generator, especially if the examiner has sound knowledge of the foot and ankle surface anatomy (Table 8.1).

Common Differential Diagnoses for Foot and Ankle Pain

1. **Tendon disorders (tendinopathy, tenosynovitis, tear)**—during the initial phase, pain from tendinopathy is usually mild in intensity, localized, intermittent and occurs with activities that require contraction of the tendon/muscle. The pain then gradually becomes constant as the condition progresses. Acute injuries from trauma or chronic overuse injuries with or without faulty biomechanics are common causes of tendon dysfunction. Patients can easily recognize the inciting event in the case of trauma; however, they may have difficulty associating subtle faulty biomechanics or overuse injuries with the underlying etiology of tendon dysfunction. Common tendon disorders in the foot and ankle include Achilles tendon on the posterior heel, posterior tibialis tendon (PTT) on the medial aspect of the hindfoot and ankle, flexor hallucis longus tendon on the posteromedial aspect, and peroneus tendon on the lateral aspect.
   I. Achilles tendinopathy: The patient typically presents with gradual onset of pain and tenderness 1 to 2 inches proximal to the insertion of the tendon. Symptoms are often aggravated by activities, such as walking and running, which require repetitive soleus muscle contraction. If the pain is located at the insertion site (posterior calcaneal tuberosity), insertional Achilles tendinopathy should be suspected.
   II. PTT dysfunction: The patient typically presents with pain and swelling on the medial hindfoot (between the medial malleolus and navicular tuberosity). Symptoms get worse with prolonged standing and walking. Insufficient posterior tibialis muscle/tendon is the most common reason for acquired flat foot (pes planus) deformity. PTT is at a mechanical disadvantage in pes planus. With the progression of the PTT dysfunction and pes planovalgus deformity, the patient may then complain of pain in the lateral hind and midfoot
2. **Bursitis**—retrocalcaneal bursa, located between the posterior calcaneal tuberosity and Achilles tendon, can cause pain that is similar to insertional Achilles tendinopathy. Bursitis pain is usually constant and worsens with external compression (often caused by tight shoes). With significant effusion, there is a loss of contour of the Achilles tendon. It is often difficult to differentiate precalcaneal bursitis (adventitial bursitis superficial to the Achilles tendon)

TABLE 8.1 ■ Musculoskeletal Pathologies Based on the Location of Pain and Maximal Tenderness

Region	Pathologies and Notes
Plantar heel	Plantar fasciitis: pain on the medial calcaneal tuberosity. Most common cause of plantar heel pain Plantar fibromatosis: palpable nodule often with tenderness, distal to the insertion of the plantar fascia Fat pad atrophy: pain after walking, frequently with a history of steroid injection to the plantar fascia Stress fracture: vague deep pain, associated with risk factors, such as osteoporosis, diabetes mellitus, longstanding steroid use, calcaneovarus, or history of a recent change inactivity Bony tumor (e.g., interosseous lipoma)[12] Peroneus longus and brevis tendinopathy/tenosynovitis/tear
Posterior heel/ ankle	Noninsertional Achilles tendinopathy/tear: Most common cause of posterior heel pain, 2–3 inches proximal to the insertion to posterior calcaneal tuberosity Insertional Achilles tendinopathy: pain at the insertion of the tendon Os trigonum syndrome: deep posterolateral pain ± h/o minor ankle injury Flexor hallucis longus tendinopathy/tenosynovitis: posterior medial hindfoot/ankle pain ± h/o ankle sprain or overuse Retrocalcaneal/superficial calcaneal bursitis: worse wearing tight shoes
Dorsal ankle	High ankle sprain (syndesmosis): persistent pain after eversion ankle sprain ± instability Anterolateral impingement syndrome: gradual onset of pain after injury, pain during the terminal stance phase of gait Osteochondritis dissecans: chronic pain after an ankle sprain. Often poorly localized Talonavicular and calcaneocuboid joint/ligament sprain or arthritis
Medial ankle/ hindfoot	Posterior tibialis tendinopathy, tear, and tenosynovitis: Most common cause of acquired flat foot, pain between the medial malleolus and navicular tuberosity. Less commonly, flexor digitorum longus tendinopathy Deltoid ligament sprain: h/o eversion injury Arthritis: local pain h/o tarsal coalition or abnormal foot alignment (pes planus, cavus)
Lateral ankle/ hindfoot	Lateral ankle ligament sprain: Most common cause of lateral ankle pain, h/o inversion injury Peroneal tendinopathy, tear, tenosynovitis, and subluxation Sinus tarsi syndrome: persistent local pain (at sinus tarsi) after ankle sprain Calcaneocuboid joint arthritis
Lateral midfoot	Cuboid-fourth metatarsal arthritis, a subluxation (cuboid subluxation ± minor trauma/ sprain), and sprain Painful os peroneal syndrome
Medial midfoot	Kohler disease (navicular osteochondrosis), Mueller Weiss syndrome (navicular osteonecrosis) Painful accessory navicular syndrome Naviculocuneiform arthritis: often associated with hypermobile cuneiform-first metatarsal joint Lisfranc injury Flexor hallucis longus or flexor digitorum longus tendinopathy or tethering of tendons
Medial forefoot	Gout: MC cause of acute nontraumatic disabling foot pain. First metatarsophalangeal (MTP) joint; MC location Hallux rigidus/limitus: pain on the dorsum of first MTP joint initially Hallux valgus with bursitis: pain on the medial side of first MTP, irritated by tight shoes Sesamoiditis, sesamoid fracture/necrosis: pain on the plantar aspect of the first MTP joint Subluxation or dislocation of second metatarsophalangeal joint Stress fracture of second metatarsal bone; often with preceding activity change Freiberg disease (osteonecrosis of second metatarsal head): more common in adolescent female
Lesser toes	Intermetatarsal bursitis ± irritation of an interdigital nerve Taylor's bunion (Bunoinette deformity) on the lateral side of fifth metatarsal head MTP joint arthritis/synovitis (highly involved in inflammatory arthropathy; underrecognized) Lateral overloading syndrome: often h/o medial arch support use

(From S.W. Lee, Musculoskeletal Injuries and Conditions: Assessment and Management, Demos Medical, New York, 2017.)

from retrocalcaneal bursitis. Precalcaneal bursitis can coexist with retrocalcaneal bursitis, and both usually are aggravated by external compression. The patient usually reports relief of pain when walking barefoot or with slippers and shoes without heel countertop.

In the lateral forefoot region, the intermetatarsal bursa can be inflamed, causing metatarsalgia. Wearing tight shoes squeezing the forefoot can aggravate the pain. Similar to the retrocalcaneal and precalcaneal bursitis, patients prefer to walk barefoot or to use slippers. The patient may also complain of sensory symptoms, such as tingling and pins/needle sensation because of the proximity of the bursa to the intermetatarsal nerve.

3. **Ligament injury (sprain)**—ankle sprain is one of the most common sports injuries and is the most common cause of ligamentous injury. It is particularly common in sports or activities that require cutting, changing direction, jumping, or tackles. The anterior talofibular ligament is the most commonly injured ligament, typically from inversion and the ankle plantarflexion mechanism. A medial ankle sprain is less common and usually requires significant trauma to occur. Occasionally, there could be bony injury involvement of the proximal fibula (Maisonneuve fracture). A high ankle sprain involves ankle syndesmosis injury, affects ankle mortise stability, and can be a source of chronic ankle pain with instability. Other ligament sprain injuries include the bifurcate ligament on the lateral midfoot and Lisfranc ligament on the medial forefoot.

4. **Stress fracture**—metatarsal bone is the most common site followed by the calcaneus. History of trauma or change of activities may be missing or underrecognized by the patient and clinician. Risk factors include diabetes, longstanding steroid use, osteoporosis, mineral bone disease, and abnormal biomechanics (including calcaneovarus). The patient often complains of deep and vague pain. Pain often worsens with heel walking in cases of calcaneal stress fracture (but is able to stand and bear weight differentiating it from a displaced fracture). The clinician has to be aware of the initial lagging of plain x-rays in revealing pathologic findings.

5. **Plantar fasciitis**—heel pain from plantar fasciitis is the most common cause of foot pain. Typically located on the plantar aspect of the heel, worse with the first few steps in the morning then gradually improves. Also it may get worse with prolonged standing and walking, especially with low heeled shoes. Tenderness is usually located at the medial tuberosity of the calcaneus or along the proximal plantar fascia.

6. **Osteoarthritis (OA)**—primary OA is relatively rare in the ankle (tibiotalar) joint. Arthropathy of the ankle joint usually involves a prior history of trauma. The most common joint involved in primary OA in the foot and ankle region is the first metatarsophalangeal joint in the forefoot accompanied by pain with standing and walking (late stance phase initially) and stiffness. It is not uncommon in the talonavicular joint at the medial hindfoot, which usually manifests as pain that is worse in the initial loading phase of stance. The pain is usually insidious in onset. Identification of different phases of gait can be useful to further localize the pathology.

7. **Fat pad atrophy**—pain and discomfort from fat pad atrophy is an underrecognized entity that mimics pain from plantar fasciitis. It can be insidious and typically occurs after repeated steroid injections (or penetrating trauma to fat pad). The patient presents with difficulty walking with the hard-soled shoes or barefoot.

8. **Rheumatoid arthritis (RA)**—frequently involves the metatarsophalangeal joint presenting initially with metatarsalgia. Later in the course, RA involves joints and tenosynovium in the hindfoot and midfoot with subsequent pain and swelling in these locations. With advanced RA disease, joint destruction and tendon rupture can occur causing foot and ankle deformity and diffuse pain. RA can be accompanied by morning stiffness with frequent involvement of other joints and systemic manifestations.

9. **Malignancy**—foot and ankle is not a common site for bony tumor or metastasis, and most tumors are usually asymptomatic or have a nonspecific presentation. Most palpable masses

in the foot and ankle are not cancerous. Therefore diagnosing tumors in the foot and ankle region may be challenging. Symptomatic patients may present with pain which can be worse during rest (supine position or at night), and systemic manifestations, such as weight loss.[2]

10. **Osteomyelitis**—if a patient with underlying risk factors, such as diabetes mellitus, vascular disease, immunocompromise, presents with a chronic nonhealing ulcer, then the suspicion for osteomyelitis should be high. It usually presents with constant pain, often no fever. WBC count is often normal but C-reactive protein (CRP) and erythrocyte sedimentation rate (ESR) are frequently elevated.

11. **Lumbosacral radiculopathy**—most commonly occurs at the L5 followed by the S1 level. It presents with low back or buttock pain radiating down to the foot (medial and dorsal in L5 and lateral aspect in S1 radiculopathy). Motor and/or sensory deficits in the distribution of the involved root can be a significant finding that supports the diagnosis. Diagnosis can be challenging in patients who only present with pain because there are a few musculoskeletal mimickers for radiculopathy. Coexisting low back pain and foot pain can be misinterpreted as lumbosacral radiculopathy because of the fact that low back pain is very common in the general population.

12. **Peripheral polyneuropathy**—sensory symptoms (pain, numbness, tingling, or pins/needles sensation) can be present along with the distribution of peripheral nerves (often distal and symmetric in peripheral polyneuropathy). Peripheral neuropathy related to diabetes can present with symptoms that start distally from the toes and gradually move proximally known as "dying-back phenomenon."

13. **Local entrapment neuropathy**—should be differentiated from lumbosacral radiculopathy and peripheral polyneuropathy. It is typically limited to the distribution of a single peripheral nerve, usually from stretching or compression of the nerve. Common entrapment neuropathies in the foot and ankle include tarsal tunnel syndrome, distal tarsal tunnel syndrome involving inferior calcaneal nerve (Baxter nerve), medial plantar neuropathy (jogger's foot), and anterior tarsal tunnel syndrome (Fig. 8.1). Baxter nerve entrapment syndrome requires particular attention because it does not have cutaneous sensory innervation; thus there are typically no cutaneous sensory symptoms such as numbness, tingling, or pins/needle sensation. It manifests with deep aching pain in the plantar aspect of the heel similar to plantar fasciitis. In recalcitrant heel pain, Baxter entrapment neuropathy should be included in the differential diagnosis (Table 8.2).

14. **Referred pain from proximal structures**—the pain from saphenous nerve irritation at the medial leg and medial knee can cause the pain in the medial foot and ankle. Patients who underwent procedures such as arthroscopic knee surgeries, injections, or saphenous vein grafting are at increased risk for iatrogenic saphenous neuropathy. Other pathologies involving the shin can also cause referred pain to the foot and ankle.

15. **Charcot neuroarthropathy**—if the patient has longstanding diabetes mellitus, clinicians should be aware of the possibility of neuroarthropathy. Other risk factors include alcoholism, leprosy, meningocele, tabes dorsalis/syphilis, and syringomyelia.[3] Because the typical pain is lacking and with the presence of peripheral neuropathy, it can be easily missed by the patient and the treating physician. Early diagnosis is important to prevent rapid progressive joint disease by limiting weight bearing. It is often difficult to differentiate from osteomyelitis which can also coexist. Concomitant peripheral neuropathy can cause sensory symptoms.

Case Discussion

This case describes the insidious onset of foot and ankle symptoms over a few months without preceding injury or trauma, indicating that the underlying etiology is likely degenerative or overuse injury with/without faulty biomechanics rather than acute trauma, vascular or rapidly progressive infectious or inflammatory process.

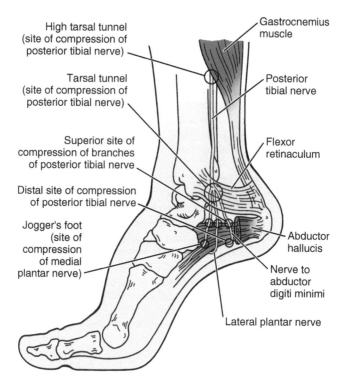

Fig. 8.1 Common locations for posterior tibial nerve entrapment (tarsal tunnel syndrome). (From D.E. Baxter, The Foot and Ankle in Sport, Mosby St Louis, 1995.)

TABLE 8.2 ■ **The Neuropathic Pain Generators Based on the Location of Pain and Sensory-Motor Deficits**

Region	Pathologies and Notes
Diffuse	Tarsal tunnel syndrome (proximal part) Distal peripheral neuropathy Lumbosacral radiculopathy (radiating pain to dorsum [L5] and lateral side of foot [S1])
Plantar	Medial • Tarsal tunnel syndrome (distal part) involving the medial plantar nerve • Medial plantar neuropathy (jogger's foot) • Medial hallucal neuropathy (at metatarsophalangeal [MTP] joint area) Lateral • Morton interdigital neuritis • Tarsal tunnel syndrome (distal part) involving the lateral plantar nerve • Lateral plantar neuropathy; neurilemma, iatrogenic, etc. Heel • Medial calcaneal N: posterior heel/cutaneous burning, pins/needles • Baxter N (first branch of the lateral plantar nerve): deep aching pain, mimicking persistent plantar fasciitis
Dorsum	Medial • Superficial peroneal neuropathy at the site perforating the crural fascia (above the ankle) • Anterior tarsal tunnel syndrome involving deep and superficial peroneal neuropathy • Hallux rigidus/limitus dorsal osteophytes irritating the deep and superficial peroneal nerves/medial dorsal branch, or the medial dorsal hallucal nerve) • Saphenous N lesion (at the knee or leg, iatrogenic injury [common cause]) • Lateral • Deep peroneal N (branch to extensor digitorum brevis, a possible cause of sinus tarsi syndrome) • Superficial peroneal N (perforating the crural fascia or distally at the navicular bone) • Sural neuralgia (lateral calcaneal branch)

N, Nerve.

(From Lee SW. *Musculoskeletal Injuries and Conditions: Assessment and Management.* NY, NY: Demos Medical; 2017.)

The gradual development of symptoms over a few months makes vascular or a rapid inflammatory process less likely underlying etiologies. Although infection is not likely the underlying etiology in this case, however, caution should always be taken in patients with risk factors.

The location of pain in the medial hindfoot can be useful information. Lack of radiating pain or pain in the knee or hip makes distant pain generators less likely. Local pathologies in this region include tendinopathies (PTT, flexor digitorum longus), bony/joint pathologies (talonavicular, naviculocuneiform joint, talus, navicular, and accessory navicular bone), and neuropathies (tibial nerve branches, such as medial plantar nerve, medial calcaneal nerve, or a proximal nerve, such as saphenous nerve).

Lack of pain radiating distally or proximally makes nerve pathologies less likely although it cannot be completely ruled out.

One way to differentiate tendon from bony or joint pathologies is to exert the tendon using body weight. If the pain is reproduced by contraction of the muscle/tendon (concentrically or eccentrically) rather than joint mobilization, then tendon pathology is more likely to be the pain generator. In contrast, pain reproduced by passive joint mobilization without tendon contraction favors joint pathology as the pain generator. However, it is not often easy to differentiate one from the other.

Osteomyelitis is less likely in this case given that there are no red flags, plain imaging findings supporting the infectious process, or elevated WBC. However, as these tests can be negative initially, physicians should consider further tests, such as ESR and CRP, and/or advanced imaging, such as magnetic resonance imaging (MRI) if clinical suspicion is high.

Charcot neuroarthropathy can be considered as a cause of acquired pes planus, but it is uncommon unless there are underlying risk factors, such as longstanding diabetes.

Objective Data

Complete blood count—within normal limits
Coagulation panel—within normal limits
Complete metabolic panel—within normal limits
ESR and CRP—within normal limits
X-ray of foot and ankle—pes planus (calcaneal pitch angle 10 degrees [normal 17–32 degrees] on lateral weight-bearing view). Osteophytes in the posterior and medial calcaneal tuberosity. Mild degenerative changes and joint space narrowing in the talonavicular joint. No sclerotic or lytic lesions were seen.
X-ray of the lumbar spine—degenerative disc disease L4–L5 and L5–S1 disc spaces narrowing, no fractures or dislocation were seen
Musculoskeletal ultrasonography—heterogeneity in the PTT and increased thickness of PTT on the right side

Further Case Discussion

The aforementioned laboratory and imaging data are helpful to further narrow down the differential diagnosis.

Several morbid conditions can be ruled out based on the objective data. Normal ESR and CRP make an infection process and osteomyelitis unlikely.

Although the absence of preceding trauma makes acute displaced fractures and dislocation less likely, stress fractures cannot be completely ruled out depending on the timing of when the initial plain radiographs are obtained (usually negative if taken within a week of symptom onset). Similarly, the absence of lytic or blastic lesions make bony tumor less likely, but cannot be completely ruled out without obtaining advanced imaging, such as MRI.

The objective data are notable for x-ray and musculoskeletal ultrasound findings suggestive of pes planus, degenerative changes in the talonavicular joint with joint space narrowing, and tibialis posterior tendinopathy.

MRI may be necessary if there is suspicion of a subcortical lesion, bony edema, nondisplaced fracture/stress fracture, or soft tissue mass that is difficult to assess with ultrasonography.

The absence of sensory or motor symptoms makes nerve conduction studies and electromyography (EMG) less useful in this case. EMG can be useful if there is suspicion of concomitant entrapment neuropathy or peripheral neuropathy involving large-diameter nerve fibers. Occasionally, chronic heel pain from Baxter entrapment neuropathy lacking cutaneous sensory or motor symptoms can be confirmed by an EMG test.

Review of Proposed Pathology and Pathobiomechanics

In closed kinetic chain activities, movements at different levels of the lower extremities (pelvis, hip, knee, ankle, foot [subtalar, midtarsal and forefoot]) are coupled. Pronation and supination is a common movement pattern that combines three-dimensional movements in sagittal, frontal, and axial planes.

During pronation, the forefoot abducts accompanied by midfoot dorsiflexion and hindfoot eversion. Tibia and femur internally rotate, and the knee moves into valgus. During supination, there are opposite movements of pronation in each lower extremity part.

Although these are normal movements that occur during walking, any excessive motion can affect the lower extremity musculoskeletal systems negatively.

Tibialis posterior inverts the hindfoot and plantar flexes the foot, therefore acts against pronation during walking. It is most active during the midstance of the gait, primarily preventing the foot from everting past the neutral position by locking the midtarsal (intersection of calcaneocuboid and talonavicular) joint.[4] Therefore insufficiency of the tibialis posterior can contribute to overpronation response resulting in hindfoot eversion, failure of locking the midtarsal joint with navicular dropping leading to pes planus deformity and decreased plantar load transfer anteriorly[5] (Fig. 8.2).

Tibialis posterior tendon is an important dynamic structure that supports the foot arch. Other contributing soft tissue structures include spring ligaments, plantar aponeurosis, peroneus muscle, gastrocsoleus muscle, and so on.[6]

Tight Achilles tendon can aggravate overpronation with increasing hindfoot eversion by pulling the posterior calcaneal tuberosity lateral to the ground reaction force.

Multiple theories exist on the development of PTT dysfunction, including degenerative, inflammatory, and microtraumatic etiologies. Hypovascularity about 4 cm proximal to the tendon insertion site can contribute to the development of degeneration of PTT. More than 50% of patients report remote histories of trauma supporting the microtraumatic theory. It is also more common in obese females, those over 40 years of age, and with a history of HTN, diabetes mellitus, and seronegative arthropathy.[7]

Typically, PTT dysfunction is a progressive condition, initially starting with tenosynovitis then progressing to elongation of the tendon and degeneration.

With the progression of PTT dysfunction, the structural deformity of the foot follows. As planus deformity progresses, secondary pain syndrome usually occurs because of the impingement of lateral foot structures (calcaneocuboid, cuboid-metatarsal joints).

Pes planus is a descriptive term, rather than a diagnosis, and can be divided into flexible or rigid forms. The flexible type may be physiologic or can be associated with certain disorders, such as ligament laxity, obesity, hypotonia, calcaneovalgus, or other conditions. The rigid type is often associated with disorders such as congenital vertical talus, tarsal coalition, peroneal spasticity, and trauma.[8]

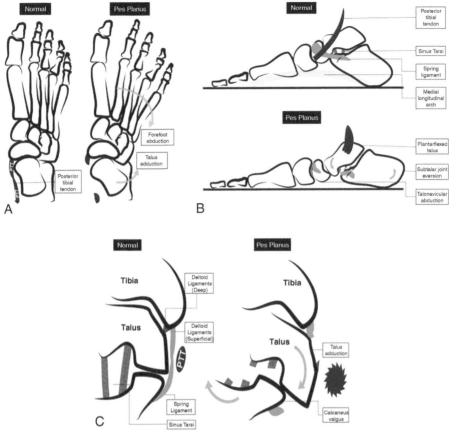

Fig. 8.2 (A) Axial, (B) sagittal, and (C) coronal plane views of normal and abnormal foot alignment with posterior tibialis dysfunction. (From Y.-C. Lin, J.Y. Kwon, M. Ghorbacnhoseini, J.S. Wu, The hindfoot arch. Radiol. Clin. N. Am. 54 (5) (2016), 951–968, Fig. 4.)

CLINICAL SIGNS AND SYMPTOMS OF POSTERIOR TIBIALIS TENDON DYSFUNCTION

Initially, the pain and swelling are minimal which causes a delay between the symptom onset and clinic encounter. The pain is typically located between the medial malleolus and navicular tuberosity and occasionally radiates to the medial calf. Swelling can accompany the pain; however, it is often difficult to be identified or recognized by patients, especially in patients with obese body habitus.

Symptoms are slowly progressive and typically are aggravated by prolonged walking and sports activities. The pain can later migrate to the lateral aspect of the foot as the pes planus deformity progresses because of the impingement of lateral hindfoot and midfoot structures.

The posterior tibial nerve and branches of the posterior tibial nerve are located in the vicinity of the PTT, which may cause the patient to have sensory symptoms or "tarsal tunnel syndrome" like symptoms secondary to increased pressure inside the flexor retinaculum with posterior tibialis tenosynovitis.

It is important to examine patients while they are barefoot with adequate exposure to the lower extremities. The alignment of the lower extremity should be examined. Pronation or hyperpronation patterns include knee valgus, tibial internal rotation, hindfoot valgus (eversion), midfoot dorsiflexion, and forefoot abduction. The pelvis may be tilted toward the ipsilateral side with functional limb shortening. In the case of forefoot abduction, the examiner may observe more toes from behind, referred to as the "too many toes" sign.

Leg length should be evaluated by measuring the distance from the umbilicus or the anterior superior iliac spine to the medial malleolus; however, accurate measurement can sometimes be technically challenging.

A functional assessment of the tibialis posterior can be done by the "heel-rise test." Initially, the double heel rise should be tested by asking the patient to raise both heels at the same time. Failure of heel inversion indicates insufficiency of PTT. If the patient is able to perform the double heel-rise test without observing a deformity, then single heel-rise test can be done by single-leg standing then raising the ipsilateral heel. Failure of heel inversion indicates PTT dysfunction. This test may be difficult to perform in patients with significant forefoot pain or balance dysfunction (Fig. 8.3).

Pain reproduced by resistive muscle contraction (hindfoot inversion and midfoot plantarflexion) can also suggest PTT mediated pain. Resisted big toe flexion and lessor toes flexion can be performed to evaluate for painful flexor hallucis longus and flexor digitorum longus tendons.

It is important to assess for concomitant heel cord tightness by performing the Silfverskiold test.

Neurologic examination is typically normal other than mild weakness during functional testing (such as heel-rise test) of PTT. It is also important to examine for possible coexisting tarsal tunnel syndrome or concomitant peripheral neuropathy.

IMAGING STUDIES

Plain radiographs are very useful in identifying any structural deformity, gross alignment, and degenerative joint disease. In the setting of trauma, the Ottawa ankle rules can be useful for reducing

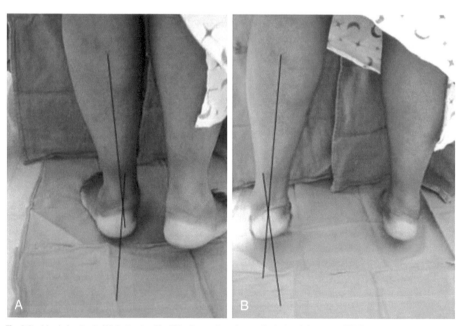

Fig. 8.3 Heel-rise test. (A) Patient with difficulty performing a single heel-rise test. (B) Patient performing double heel-rise test with hindfoot inversion. (From J. Hix, C. Kim, R.W. Mendicino, K. Saltrick, A.R. Catanzariti, Calcaneal osteotomies for the treatment of adult-acquired flatfoot, Clin. Podiatr. Med. Surg. 24 (4) (2007) 699–719.)

unnecessary imaging.[9] If the patient has tenderness at the medial or lateral malleolus, the base of fifth metatarsal or navicular bone, or is unable to bear weight for at least four steps, then x-ray imaging can be very useful with high sensitivity to abnormal findings.

In standing anteroposterior (AP) x-ray, signs that are suggestive of pes planus include talocalcaneal angle greater than 35 degrees, increased angle of talus and first metatarsal, heel valgus, and talonavicular uncoverage. In the lateral weight-bearing view, the angle between the long axis of the talus and long axis of the first metatarsal (Meary angle) can be measured and suggests pes planus if more than 4 degrees convex downwards. Calcaneal pitch line (inclination angle, normal 17–32 degrees) between the ground and the line along the inferior border of the calcaneus is also frequently used to document pes planus when decreased and pes cavus when increased.

The accessory navicular bone is not uncommon, 2% to 14% depending on the study. It can be a source of medial arch pain and x-ray imaging with a 45-degree eversion oblique view is necessary for evaluation. There is no causal relationship between pes planus and accessory navicular bone, but PTT dysfunction may correlate with accessory navicular bony injury.

It is important to know that findings of plain radiographs are typically normal in the early stage of PTT dysfunction.

Because the PTT is a soft tissue structure, ultrasonography (US) or MRI can be very useful for direct evaluation of the PTT. Typical US findings in PTT dysfunction include tenosynovial effusion, increased heterogeneity, increased tendon thickness, and increased vascularity of the tissue. Inexperienced examiners may take the granulation tissue filling the gap of ruptured PTT or remaining flexor digitorum longus tendon (FDLT) as intact PTT tendon. Loss of fibrillar pattern in the long axis view and "broomstick" appearance in a short-axis view are useful findings to differentiate the tendon from the granulation tissue.

MRI is the best imaging method overall for evaluating the foot and ankle musculoskeletal disorders; however, the lack of correlation of pain, function, and imaging findings should be recognized, especially in the elderly population. MRI findings in PTT dysfunction typically illustrate increased T2 signal intensity in tenosynovitis or tendon tears. It can also evaluate any intracortical bony lesion such as avascular necrosis (Muller-Weiss, Freiberg disease), osteochondrosis (Kohler disease), bony tumor, nondisplaced stress fracture (early stage), and ligament sprain or tear.

ELECTROMYOGRAPHY

EMG can be used to evaluate for possible concomitant peripheral neuropathy, lumbosacral radiculopathy, or focal entrapment neuropathy.

Routine sensory nerve conduction studies (such as sural and superficial peroneal nerves) can be useful to identify distal sensory peripheral neuropathy and to differentiate preganglionic versus postganglionic lesions. Plantar (medial and lateral) nerve conduction studies may increase sensitivity in distal peripheral neuropathy as the segment (plantar nerve) being measured in the foot is more distal than the sural nerve (measured in the ankle). However, the lack of response in the asymptomatic older population (age ≥65 years) and a relatively wide variation of normal parameters based on age and height can make interpretation challenging.

Hoffmann reflex study can be useful in S1 radiculopathy and early detection of peripheral polyneuropathy; however, limitations are similar to the sensory nerve condition study (often unobtainable in a normal person age ≥65 years).

Motor nerve conduction study and needle EMG can be useful to determine prognosis if there is a significant weakness. Significantly reduced amplitude and discrete motor unit recruitment patterns indicate poor prognosis.

Because needle EMG can test muscles innervated by different branches of the tibial nerve (medial plantar, lateral plantar, and inferior calcaneal branches), it can be very useful in the evaluation of focal entrapment neuropathy, such as tarsal tunnel syndrome, medial plantar neuropathy (jogger's foot), lateral plantar neuropathy, and Baxter entrapment neuropathy (inferior calcaneal neuropathy).

DISCUSSION

Morbid conditions such as infectious conditions, Charcot neuroarthropathy, progressive inflammatory arthropathy, or tumors should be suspected if red flags are present, which necessitate timely investigation and early aggressive management. If morbid conditions are ruled out, then conservative management can be considered for initial treatment.

Tight Achilles tendon is common in the aging population and has a negative impact on the PTT advancing pes planus. Therefore it is important to address the tightness of the Achilles tendon early in the course of management by stretching the gastrocnemius muscle. Stretching the gastrocsoleus muscle (of Achilles muscle-tendon complex) should be done in an extended knee position, rather than flexed knee position which only stretches the soleus muscle. To decrease subtalar compensation that mitigates Achilles stretching, slight forefoot adduction is necessary to limit the midtarsal and subtalar joints mobility.

To reduce the impact of a tight heel cord on the subtalar joint (promoting pronation response), a heel lift can be considered temporarily. A heel lift can reduce loading on the PTT, as well as reduce the compensatory response of the tight heel cord. A medial heel wedge with extension (medial posting) can be added to accommodate forefoot varus secondary to hindfoot eversion.

If a patient wears worn-out shoes (commonly medial outsole), it should be replaced with a new roomier shoe. Patients tend to choose tighter shoes that they used to wear before the development of PTT dysfunction. PTT dysfunction with gradual loss of longitudinal and transverse arch makes the patient's foot longer and wider. Patients should be educated about the importance of changing their shoes to newer ones that should have room for the possible addition of in-shoe inserts or orthosis. Using roomier shoes, however, may be challenging among patients with balance dysfunction.

In the case of tenosynovitis of PTT, Unna boot dressing can be applied for 1 to 2 weeks and can be repeated two to three times. An Unna boot is a semirigid dressing impregnated with zinc and glycine. It has been used traditionally to control edema secondary to venous insufficiency or early stage of lymphedema. It decreases swelling and provides relative rest on the PTT without interfering physical activity.

Orthosis

Because PTT dysfunction has a progressive nature, clinicians can consider aggressive intervention in the early stages, including prescribing the University of California Biomechanical Laboratory (UCBL) orthotic to support subtalar neutral alignment and mitigate hyperpronation and navicular collapse (Fig. 8.4). UCBL may not be sturdy enough to be used in obese patients. In this case, supramalleolar orthosis (SMO) or Arizona ankle-foot orthosis (AFO) can be considered. Arizona AFO is a more effective orthosis than UCBL and SMO in controlling subtalar joint and ankle joint movements; however, it is the least tolerated by patients because of its bulky design. Patient compliance is important for the best outcome. Physiatrists should be able to address common problems associated with using the orthoses and should be in close communication with the orthotist.

Physical Therapy

A course of physical therapy, including education of gastrocnemius stretching, strengthening of ankle inverters, toe flexors (intrinsic and extrinsic), and dynamic balance exercise can be tried.

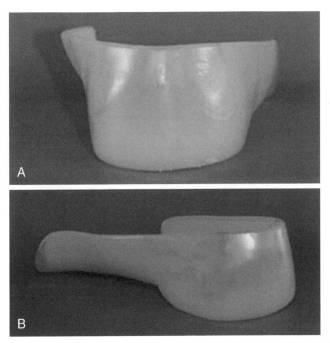

Fig. 8.4 University of California Biomechanics Laboratory insert. (A) Posterior view. (B) Medial view. (From L.B. Chou, K.L. Wapner, Conservative Treatment of the Foot. Mann's Surgery of the Foot and Ankle, 9e, Saunders, Philadelphia, 2014, Fig. 4.4A and B.)

Intrinsic foot muscle exercise is increasingly emphasized as part of the foot core system exercise.[10] Several methods are suggested, including towel curls, marble pick-ups, short foot exercise/foot doming, etc. Although the efficacy of physical therapy is challenged in its direct benefit on PTT dysfunction, there is no doubt that it is beneficial for overall lower extremity musculoskeletal problems.

Pharmacotherapy and Injection

A short course of nonsteroidal antiinflammatory drugs can be tried, but caution is required to prevent adverse effects. Anticonvulsants and tricyclic antidepressants may be tried if there are concomitant sensory symptoms, such as tingling and pins/needles sensation. Narcotic analgesics and muscle relaxants are rarely indicated in patients with PTT dysfunction.

Steroid injections should be tried with caution as PTT is a weight-bearing structure. In the early stage with tenosynovitis, imaging (ultrasonography) guided injection can be tried into the tenosynovium, but repeated steroid injections are strongly discouraged because of the concerns for tendon rupture.

Referral to Surgery

If a patient fails to respond to nonoperative therapy after at least a few months with disabling symptoms, then a surgical referral can be considered. Surgical options include tenosynovectomy, primary repair, medial calcaneal osteotomy, gastrocnemius recess, tendon transfer, triple arthrodesis, and lateral column lengthening. If there is an acute rupture of the PTT, surgical referral should not be delayed.

Summary

A patient presented with chronic foot and ankle pain, particularly in the medial hindfoot. She demonstrated symptoms and signs suggestive of PTT dysfunction. The patient was found to have pes planus as well. Further evaluation included x-ray and ultrasound imaging which confirmed the diagnosis. Subsequently, she was educated on wearing roomier shoes, the use of heel lift inserts, and starting a home exercise program focusing on gastrocnemius stretching. At 4 weeks follow-up, she reported only mild improvement and was then referred for 4 weeks of physical therapy consisting of short foot exercise (intrinsic foot muscle strengthening), gradual resistive strengthening exercise of the PTT, continuation of gastrocnemius stretching, and neuromuscular training exercise. Custom made UCBL foot orthosis was also prescribed.

At a follow-up visit 3 months later, the patient reported resolution of pain, and she did not report any problem using the UCBL orthosis. There was no progression of pes planus clinically nor were there PTT pathologies in-office ultrasound evaluation. She continued to be compliant with the home exercise program.

Key Points

- Underlying etiologies of foot and ankle pain are diverse and classified into musculoskeletal versus neuropathic and regional versus distant pain generators. The structural approach is useful to differentiate complex etiologies.
- Careful attention should be placed on all elements of history and examination, including the location of the pain, tenderness, evaluation of biomechanics, provocating tests, and functional tests.
- Treatment options should be tailored to individual patients, including education, bracing, therapeutic exercise, precise injections, or surgical referral.

CLINICAL PEARLS

Tibialis posterior tendon (PTT) is an important dynamic stabilizer that supports the foot arch, and the insufficiency of PTT is the most common cause of acquired flatfoot. Diagnosis is made based on clinical evaluation (tenderness in medial hindfoot, heel-rise test, deformity) and ultrasonography (and/or MRI) can confirm the structural pathology. Orthosis for PTT dysfunction includes University of California Biomechanical Laboratory orthosis, supramalleolar orthosis, and Arizona ankle-foot orthosis.

References

1. R.E. Cortina, B.L. Morris, B.G. Vopat, Gastrocnemius recession for metatarsalgia, Foot Ankle Clin. 23 (1) (2018) 57–68.
2. N.O. Murai, O. Teniola, W.L. Wang, B. Amini, Bone and soft tissue tumors about the foot and ankle, Radiol. Clin. North Am. 56 (6) (2018) 917–934.
3. J.C. Stanley, A.M. Collier, Charcot osteo-arthropathy, Curr. Orthop. 22 (6) (2008) 428–433.
4. G.C. Pomeroy, R.H. Pike, T.C. Beals, A. Manoli 2nd, Acquired flatfoot in adults due to dysfunction of the posterior tibial tendon, J. Bone Joint Surg. Am. 81 (8) (1999) 1173–1182.
5. D.W. Wong, Y. Wang, A.K. Leung, M. Yang, M. Zhang, Finite element simulation on posterior tibial tendinopathy: load transfer alteration and implications to the onset of pes planus, Clin. Biomech. (Bristol, Avon) 51 (2018) 10–16.
6. D.H. Richie Jr., Biomechanics and clinical analysis of the adult acquired flatfoot, Clin. Podiatr. Med. Surg. 24 (4) (2007) 617–644 vii.

7. G.B. Holmes Jr., R.A. Mann, Possible epidemiological factors associated with rupture of the posterior tibial tendon, Foot Ankle 13 (2) (1992) 70–79.
8. S.E. Yagerman, M.B. Cross, R. Positano, S.M. Doyle, Evaluation and treatment of symptomatic pes planus, Curr. Opin. Pediatr. 23 (1) (2011) 60–67.
9. J. Heyworth, Ottawa ankle rules for the injured ankle, BMJ 326 (7386) (2003) 405–406.
10. P.O. McKeon, J. Hertel, D. Bramble, I. Davis, The foot core system: a new paradigm for understanding intrinsic foot muscle function, Br. J. Sports Med. 49 (5) (2014).
11. S.W. Lee, Musculoskeletal Injuries and Conditions: Assessment and Management, Demos Medical: New York, 2017.
12. T. Propeck, M.A. Bullard, J. Lin, K. Doi, W. Martel, Radiologic-pathologic correlation of intraosseous lipomas, AJR Am. J. Roentgenol. 175 (3) (2000) 673–678.

CHAPTER 9

Fibromyalgia

Dr. Kishan A. Sitapara, MD ■ Dr. Michelle Stern, MD

Case Presentation

A 47-year-old female presents to the Physical Medicine and Rehabilitation (PM&R) clinic with increasing fatigue and pain in both of her shoulders, hips, back, and arms for 8 months. Patient reports that the pain started precipitously. Reports that "everything hurts" and that she feels "tired all the time." States that the pain seems to be in her muscles and does not necessarily feel pain in her joints. Pain is a constant, dull, throbbing, 7/10 pain that does not really improve with nonsteroidal antiinflammatory drugs (NSAIDs), ice, acetaminophen. Notes that sometimes a heating pad seems to help the pain but that it only helps for small amounts of time. Pain interferes with her sleep and is worse in the mornings and before bed. Denies any changes in her mood and states that she normally is happy but over the last several months the constant pain is making her less upbeat. States she is too busy to exercise and that she is usually sedentary during the workday. Denies any nausea, vomiting, diarrhea, shortness of breath, swelling of her joints, joint stiffness, weight loss, difficulty breathing, fevers, chills, or recent cough.

Past medical history: Obesity, hypertension.

Past surgical history: Cholecystectomy.

Allergies: Shellfish.

Medications: Ibuprofen as needed, acetaminophen as needed, lisinopril 20 mg daily.

Social history: Lives with her three children and husband in a third-floor walk-up building. Works as a receptionist. Drinks about 1 to 2 glasses of wine weekly. Denies any current or past cigarette or illicit drug use.

BP: 145/85 mmHg, PR: 88 per min, RR: 16/min, pulse oxygenation: 98% on room air, Temp: 98.8° F, BMI: 35 kg/m^2.

General: Mild distress, appears tired and uncomfortable. Slightly withdrawn.

Head, eyes, ears, nose, throat: Normocephalic. Pupils equal, reactive to light. Extraocular muscles intact. Sclera nonicteric. Moist oral mucosa.

Neck: Supple. Thyroid nonenlarged, no goiter appreciated.

Lungs: Breathing comfortably on room air. Clear to auscultation bilaterally, no wheezing, rales, rhonchi.

Cardiovascular: Regular rate and rhythm with no murmurs, rubs, gallops.

Abdomen: Obese, soft, nontender. Bowel sounds present in all four quadrants.

Extremities: Trace bilateral, nonpitting pedal edema.

Musculoskeletal: Passive and active range of motion mostly within normal limits in all four extremities, with some voluntary resistance secondary to reported pain on terminal bilateral shoulder flexion and initial shoulder abduction. Active range of motion decreased on forward flexion at the waist. Tenderness noted on palpation over bilateral deltoids, biceps, quadriceps, gastrocnemii. Tenderness noted over bilateral sternocleidomastoid, splenius capitus, and trapezius.

NEUROLOGIC:

Manual muscle testing 4/5 bilaterally on shoulder abduction, shoulder flexion, hip flexion. 5/5 bilaterally on elbow flexion, elbow extension, finger flexion, finger extension, knee flexion, knee extension, dorsiflexion, plantar flexion, great toe flexion, and great toe extension.

Sensation grossly intact to light touch.

Labs: Complete blood count (CBC): white blood cell (WBC): 7.8 x 10^9/L, Hgb: 13.2g/dL, HCT 40%, platelets 230 x 10^9/L.

Erythrocyte sedimentation rate (ESR): 13 mm/h.

Imaging: No prior imaging available.

Discussion

Fibromyalgia (FM) is a chronic functional illness that presents with widespread musculoskeletal pain, as well as a constellation of symptoms, including fatigue, cognitive dysfunction, sleep difficulties, stiffness, anxiety, and depressed mood.[1] It is the most common cause of chronic widespread musculoskeletal pain.[2] Fibromyalgia's prevalence in the United States is between 2% and 8% of the general population with women being diagnosed with the illness 2:1 as compared with men.[3,4] The average age of onset is between the ages of 30 and 50 years.[6] Risk factors include female gender, lower educational status, lower household income, history of disability, and middle age.[5]

Because of the nature of disease, where patients experience invalidation by medical services, their families and societies regarding the recognition and management of disease, direct, indirect, and immeasurable costs are considerable.[6] FM patients make 10 to 18 primary care appointments per year and are hospitalized on average once every 3 years.[6–10] Patients also reported missing 0.4 to 3.0 days from work and being unable to complete 3.6 to 35.4 hours of unpaid informal work because of FM, including child care, housework, yard work, or other daily activities.[6,10]

The mean annual cost per patient ranged from US \$2274 to \$9573 or even more in various studies depending on the severity of symptoms and rout of cost calculation.[6,8,10,11] Overall, it seems the clinical and economic burden of the disease on societies is so high that FM is on the same level as other chronic diseases, such as diabetes or hypertension; however, the latter usually receives much more attention from the healthcare and nonhealthcare systems.[6,12,13]

SYMPTOMS

Pain is the most common reported symptom of FM. The pain reported can be described as chronic, deep, widespread, aching, radiating, shooting, or tender.[14] However, in addition to pain other symptoms are also present. The National Fibromyalgia Association conducted a survey in which people with FM reported their symptoms as shown in Fig. 9.1.

DIFFERENTIAL DIAGNOSIS

Because of the various presentations of FM and the multiple associated comorbidities, diagnosis can often be a challenge.[14] Several disorders can also mimic FM, such as hypothyroidism and inflammatory rheumatic diseases.[14] In addition, some medications may contribute to pain, such as statins, aromatase inhibitors, bisphosphonates, and opioids (i.e., opioid-induced hyperalgesia).[14] However, these conditions and many others (e.g., rheumatoid arthritis, osteoarthritis, systemic lupus erythematosus [SLE], spinal stenosis, neuropathies, Ehlers Danlos syndrome, sleep disorders [e.g., sleep apnea], and mood and anxiety disorders) also cooccur in patients with FM.[14–16]

Table 9.1 summarizes some of the key medical disorders considered in the differential diagnosis of FM that require additional assessment, tests, and specific treatment.[14]

DIAGNOSTIC CRITERIA

Because of the sometimes vague presentation of FM, it can frequently be difficult to diagnose. A 2018 study showed that the mean total time to diagnose fibromyalgia after initial presentation was 6.42 years.[17] Patients who presented with other comorbidities, at a younger age, or to an older physician were associated with an even longer time to diagnosis.[17]

The definition of FM continues to evolve reflecting the changes in understanding and shifts in diagnostic criteria. The American College of Rheumatology (ACR) 1990 diagnostic criteria required the presence of pain on both sides of the body and above and below the waist present for at least 3 months, with the presence of at least 11 of a possible 18 tender points and not

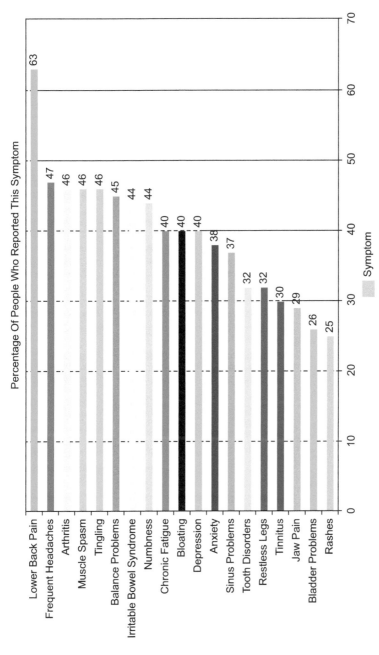

Fig. 9.1 According to a survey conducted by the National Fibromyalgia Association, this figure shows the percentage of patients with fibromyalgia who report the symptoms stated. (From R. Bennett, J. Jones, D.C. Turk, I.J. Russell, L. Matallana, An internet survey of 2,596 people with fibromyalgia. BMC Musculoskelet Disord. 8 (2007) 27.)

TABLE 9.1 ■ Summary of Some Key Medical Disorders That Should Be Considered in the Differential Diagnosis of Fibromyalgia

Medical Disorder	Differentiating Key Disorders From Fibromyalgia Differentiating Signs and Symptoms
Rheumatologic	
Rheumatoid arthritis	Predominant joint pain, symmetric joint swelling, joint line tenderness, morning stiffness >1 hour
Systemic lupus erythematosus	Multisystem involvement, joint/muscle pain, rash, photosensitivity, fever
Polyarticular osteoarthritis	Joint stiffness, crepitus, multiple painful joints
Polymyalgia rheumatica	Proximal shoulder and hip girdle pain, weakness, stiffness, more common in the elderly
Polymyositis or other myopathies	Symmetric, proximal muscle weakness, and pain
Spondyloarthropathy	Localization of spinal pain to specific sites in the neck, midthoracic, anterior chest wall, or lumbar regions, objective limitation of spinal mobility because of pain and stiffness
Osteomalacia	Diffuse bone pain, fractures, proximal myopathy with muscle weakness
Neurologic	
Neuropathy	Shooting or burning pain, tingling, numbness, weakness
Multiple sclerosis	Visual changes (unilateral partial or complete loss, double vision), ascending numbness in a leg or bandlike truncal numbness, slurred speech (dysarthria)
Infectious	
Lyme disease	Rash, arthritis or arthralgia, occurs in areas of endemic disease
Hepatitis	Right upper quadrant pain, nausea, decreased appetite
Endocrine	
Hyperparathyroidism	Increased thirst and urination, kidney stones, nausea/vomiting, decreased appetite, thinning bones, constipation
Cushing syndrome	Hypertension, diabetes, hirsutism, moon facies, weight gain
Addison disease	Postural hypotension, nausea, vomiting, skin pigmentation, weight loss
Hypothyroidism	Cold intolerance, mental slowing, constipation, weight gain, hair loss

better explained by any other disorder.[18] The newer 2010 ACR diagnostic criteria define FM as a chronic widespread pain condition associated with fatigue, sleep and cognitive disturbance, and a variety of somatic symptoms.[19,20]

The 2010 ACR diagnostic criteria focus on measurement of symptom severity and no longer rely on tender point examination.[5] Instead, many other symptoms were promoted as key features of FM.[3,4,20] These include fatigue, cognitive symptoms, and somatic symptoms. The 2010 criteria rely on a series of questions based on the Widespread Pain Index (WPI) and Symptom Severity (SS) scale.[20] According to this new ACR "Proposed Criteria," FM is defined as:

WPI score of 7 or higher and SS score of 5 or higher or WPI of 3–6 or higher and SS score of 9 or higher[20]

Symptoms remaining at approximately that level for 3 months[20]

The patient having no disorder that would otherwise explain the pain[20]

The areas of pain include:

Shoulder girdle (left), shoulder girdle (right), upper arm (left), upper arm (right), lower arm (left), lower arm (right), hip (buttock, trochanter, [left]), hip (buttock, trochanter, [right]), upper leg (left), upper leg (right), lower leg (left), lower leg (right), jaw (left), jaw (right), chest, abdomen, upper back, lower back, and neck.[20]

DIAGNOSTIC EVALUATION

History

A thorough history should always be taken. Questions emphasizing the nature, duration, and location of the pain should be asked. Associated signs and symptoms should also be addressed, including questions regarding sleep, fatigue, and mental and physical energy. Cognitive disturbances, mood disorders and other psychiatric conditions, and other conditions that overlap with FM and may be considered to be part of the diagnostic spectrum.[2] These include symptoms of chronic migraine or other headache disorders, irritable bowel syndrome, chronic pelvic and/or bladder pain, and chronic temporomandibular pain.[2]

Physical Examination

A thorough physical examination should be performed, with particular attention to a careful joint and neurologic examination to identify generalized widespread soft tissue tenderness and to exclude other illness presenting with similar symptoms.[2] The examination should include palpating multiple soft tissue and joint sites, and a joint examination should always be done, looking for any synovitis and also palpating for tenderness over the joints themselves.[2] In general, many soft tissue sites are very tender with modest palpation and are more tender than the joints.[2] There should be no soft tissue or joint swelling or redness.[2]

Laboratory Testing

There is no diagnostic laboratory test or radiographic or pathologic finding for FM. Thus testing should be kept to a minimum.[2]

As such, laboratory testing is generally unremarkable but necessary to rule out other diseases. Basic laboratory tests, such as CBC and ESR or C-reactive protein (CRP) should be collected.[21]

CBC and ESR or CRP for initial laboratory evaluation is helpful. Because FM is not an inflammatory condition, normal acute phase reactants immediately provide confidence that an occult inflammatory disorder is unlikely.[2]

Serologic tests, such as antinuclear antibody and rheumatoid factor, should be obtained only if the history and physical examination suggest an inflammatory, systemic rheumatic disease. These tests are often positive in otherwise healthy people and have very poor predictive value unless there is significant clinical suspicion of a systemic rheumatic disease.[22]

IMAGING

Like laboratory testing, imaging is done primarily to exclude an associated disease or another illness that may mimic FM, because FM itself does not cause any abnormalities in routine imaging.[2]

Treatment

Although there is no cure for FM, treatment can still be very beneficial. Treatment should be multidisciplinary and focus on improving functional activities and quality of life and on decreasing pain and other associated symptoms.[5] Because of the heterogeneity of symptoms and the poorly known pathogenesis, the therapy of FM remains a challenge.[23]

Fig. 9.2 shows treatment approaches available for patients with FM.[19]

Nonpharmacologic Treatment

According to the European League Against Rheumatism (EULAR) guidelines, once the diagnosis of FM is made, priority should be given to nonpharmacologic treatment.[21] The reason lies

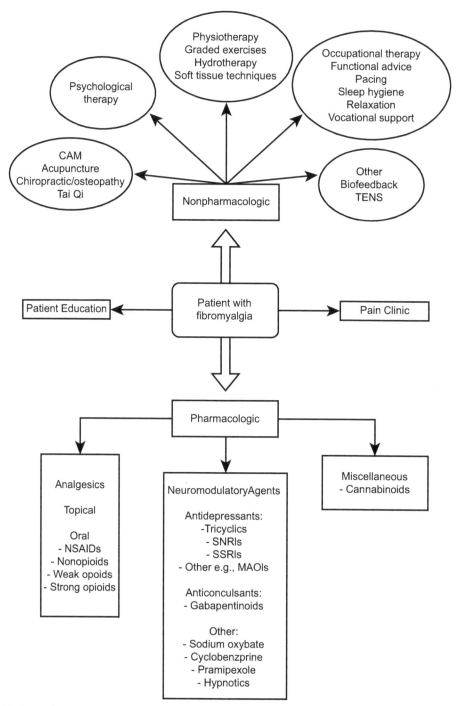

Fig. 9.2 This figure shows treatment approaches available for patients with fibromyalgia. (From H. Cohen, Controversies and challenges in fibromyalgia: a review and a proposal, Ther Adv Musculoskelet Dis. 9 (5) (2017) 115–127.)

in cost effectiveness, patient's preference, safety, and availability.[23] Physical exercise has the best profile of efficacy and safety; it should be prescribed to every patient with a diagnosis of FM.[23] A 2019 study conducted primarily with women with diagnosed FM reinforced the understanding that exercise can reduce symptoms of FM and suggests that patients who practice physical exercise have a better quality of life, with fewer depressive symptoms and absences from work, and better sense of wellbeing.[24] Furthermore, a study in 2017 looking at aerobic exercise (defined as exercises such as walking and swimming that cause harder breathing and faster heart rate than occur at rest) training for adults with FM showed that when compared with control, moderate-quality evidence indicates that aerobic exercise probably improves health-related quality of life (HRQL) and all-cause withdrawal, and low-quality evidence suggests that aerobic exercise may slightly decrease pain intensity, may slightly improve physical function, and may lead to little difference in fatigue and stiffness. Outcomes in HRQL, physical function, and pain reached clinical significance.[25] Long-term effects, however, of aerobic exercise may include little or no difference in pain, physical function, and all-cause withdrawal.[25] Despite physical exercise being a cornerstone in the nonpharmacologic management of FM, specific interventions and programs are poorly defined.[26]

Other nonpharmacologic treatment modalities may include patient education, electrotherapy, cryotherapy, and therapeutic heat.[27] Psychological intervention is a necessary component in a rehabilitation program for FM.[27] Some treatment modalities include cognitive behavioral therapy (CBT), relaxation training, group therapy, biofeedback, and stress management.[27] CBT has the best evidence of the psychological methods in FM.[5] It improves one's ability to cope with pain, reduces depressed mood, decreases healthcare-seeking behavior, and improves self-efficacy by promoting more positive, adaptive thoughts and behaviors (Evidence level 1A).[5]

Case studies have shown trigger point injections, acupuncture, tai chi, yoga, and chiropractic manipulation to reduce FM pain although evidence is limited.[5,28]

Pharmacologic Treatment

The aim is to provide a balance of medications that help the patient cope with symptoms, complementing the nonpharmacologic therapies and patient education.[19] The evidence base is poor, and patient expectations should be managed because although a symptom-based medication approach may ameliorate symptoms, it will not "cure" the pain.[19] Medications will require cautious dose escalation and monitoring of short- and long-term side effects, and discontinuation of ineffective drugs or those with intolerable side effects.[19] Table 9.2 summarizes the pharmacologic therapies useful in the treatment of FM.

CLINICAL PEARLS

Diagnostic criteria no longer requires tender points.
No diagnostic testing available to diagnose FM, only to rule out other possibilities on the differential.
Treatment requires a true multidisciplinary approach.

Summary

Fibromyalgia (FM) is a chronic, functional illness that presents with widespread musculoskeletal pain as well as a constellation of symptoms, including fatigue, cognitive dysfunction, sleep difficulties, stiffness, anxiety, and depressed mood.[1] It is the most common cause of chronic widespread musculoskeletal pain.[2] Fibromyalgia's prevalence in the United States is between 2% and 8% of the general population, with women being diagnosed with the illness 2:1 as compared to men.[4,5] Pain is the most common reported symptom of FM. Although there is no cure for FM, treatment can still be very beneficial. Treatment should be multidisciplinary and focus on improving

TABLE 9.2 ■ Pharmacologic Therapies Useful in the Treatment of Fibromyalgia

Treatment	Cost	Specifics	Evidence Level	Adverse Effects	Clinical Pearls
Pharmacologic therapies		Pharmacologic therapy is best chosen on the basis of the predominant symptoms and initiated in low dose with slow dose escalation	Level 5, consensus		Some practitioners find that getting patients on a drug regimen that helps improve symptoms before initiating nonpharmacologic therapies can help improve adherence
Tricyclic compounds		Amitriptyline, 10–70 mg every night at bedtime Cyclobenzaprine, 5–20 mg every night at bedtime	1, A	Dry mouth, weight gain, constipation, and "groggy" or drugged feeling	When effective, they can improve a wide range of symptoms including pain, sleep, and bowel and bladder syndromes Taking these drugs several hours before bedtime improves the adverse effect profile
Serotonin norepinephrine reuptake inhibitors	Duloxetine is generic, but milnacipran is not	Duloxetine, 30–120 mg/d Milnacipran, 100–200 mg/d	1, A	Nausea, palpitations, headache, fatigue, tachycardia, and hypertension	Warning patients about transient nausea, taking with food, and slowly increasing dose can increase tolerability Milnacipran might be slightly more noradrenergic than duloxetine and thus potentially more helpful for fatigue and memory problems, but also more likely to cause hypertension
Gabapentinoids	Gabapentin is generic, but pregabalin is not	Gabapentin, 800–2400 mg/d in divided doses Pregabalin, up to 600 mg/d in divided doses	1, A	Sedation, weight gain, and dizziness	Giving most or all of the dose at bedtime can increase tolerability
γ-Hydroxybutyrate	Available for treating narcolepsy and cataplexy	4.5–6.0 g every night in divided doses	1, A	Sedation, respiratory depression, and death	Shown to be efficacious but not approved by the US Food and Drug Administration because of safety concerns
Low-dose naltrexone	Low	4.5 mg/d	2 small single-center randomized controlled trials		

Cannabinoids	Not applicable	Nabilone, 0.5 mg po qhs to 1.0 mg bid	1, A	Sedation, dizziness, and dry mouth	No synthetic cannabinoid is approved in the United States for the treatment of pain
Selective serotonin reuptake inhibitors (SSRIs)	SSRIs that should be used in fibromyalgia (see Pearls) are all generic	Fluoxetine, sertraline, and paroxetine	1, A	Nausea, sexual dysfunction, weight gain, and sleep disturbance	Older, less selective SSRIs may have some efficacy in improving pain, especially at higher doses that have more prominent noradrenergic effects. Newer SSRIs (citalopram, escitalopram, and desvenlafaxine) are less effective or ineffective as analgesics
Nonsteroidal antiinflammatory drugs		No evidence of efficacy. Can be helpful to treat comorbid "peripheral pain generators"	5, D	Gastrointestinal, renal, and cardiac adverse effects	Use the lowest dose for the shortest period of time to reduce adverse effects
Opioids		Tramadol with or without acetaminophen, 50–100 mg every 6 h. No evidence of efficacy for stronger opioids	5, D	Sedation, addiction, tolerance, and opioid-induced hyperalgesia	There is increasing evidence that opioids are less effective in treating chronic pain than previously thought and that their risk-benefit profile is worse than that of other classes of analgesics

(From D.J. Clauw. Fibromyalgia and related conditions. Mayo Clin Proc. 90 (5) (2015) 680–692.)

functional activities and quality of life and on decreasing pain and other associated symptoms.[6] Due to the heterogeneity of symptoms and the poorly known pathogenesis, the therapy of FM remains a challenge.[24]

Key Points

- Fibromyalgia has a wide range of symptoms.
- Prevalence is between 2% and 8% of the general population in the United States.
- Obtaining a thorough history and physical is of the utmost importance when diagnosing FM.
- There are no diagnostic laboratory tests or radiographic or pathologic findings in FM.
- Treatment options include both nonpharmacologic and pharmacologic options.

References

1. D. Goldenberg, Diagnosis and differential diagnosis of fibromyalgia, Am. J. Med. 122 (Suppl. 12) (2009) S14–S21.
2. D. Goldenberg, P. Schur, P. Romain, Clinical manifestations and diagnosis of fibromyalgia in adults, UpToDate (2019).
3. D.J. Clauw, Fibromyalgia and related conditions, Mayo Clin. Proc. 90 (5) (2015) 680–692.
4. D.J. Clauw, Fibromyalgia: a clinical review, J. Am. Med. Assoc. 311 (15) (2014) 1547–1555.
5. M. Davies, C. Ward, J. Singh, Fibromyalgia, PM&R KnowledgeNow (2017).
6. B. Ghavidel-Parsa, A. Bidari, A. Maafi, B. Ghalebaghi, The iceberg nature of fibromyalgia burden: the clinical and economic aspects, Korean J. Pain (2015) 169–176.
7. A. Berger, E. Dukes, S. Martin, J. Edelsberg, G. Oster, Characteristics and healthcare costs of patients with fibromyalgia syndrome, Int. J. Clin. Pract. 61 (2007) 1498–1508.
8. R.L. Robinson, H.G. Birnbaum, M.A. Morley, T. Sisitsky, P.E. Greenberg, A.J. Claxton, Economic cost and epidemiological characteristics of patients with fibromyalgia claims, J. Rheumatol. 30 (2003) 1318–1325.
9. A. Berger, A. Sadosky, E. Dukes, S. Martin, J. Edelsberg, G. Oster, Characteristics and patterns of healthcare utilization of patients with fibromyalgia in general practitioner settings in Germany, Curr. Med. Res. Opin. 24 (2008) 2489–2499.
10. A. Chandran, C. Schaefer, K. Ryan, R. Baik, M. McNett, G. Zlateva, The comparative economic burden of mild, moderate, and severe fibromyalgia: results from a retrospective chart review and cross-sectional survey of working-age U.S. adults, J. Manag. Care Pharm. 18 (2012) 415–426.
11. A. Winkelmann, S. Perrot, C. Schaefer, et al., Impact of fibromyalgia severity on health economic costs: results from a European cross-sectional study, Appl. Health Econ. Health Policy 9 (2011) 125–136.
12. Y. Doron, R. Peleg, A. Peleg, L. Neumann, D. Buskila, The clinical and economic burden of fibromyalgia compared with diabetes mellitus and hypertension among Bedouin women in the Negev, Fam. Pract. 21 (2004) 415–419.
13. S. Silverman, E.M. Dukes, S.S. Johnston, N.A. Brandenburg, A. Sadosky, D.M. Huse, The economic burden of fibromyalgia: comparative analysis with rheumatoid arthritis, Curr. Med. Res. Opin. 25 (2009) 829–840.
14. L. Arnold, R. Bennett, L. Crofford, L. Dean, D. Clauw, D. Goldenberg, et al., AAPT diagnostic criteria for fibromyalgia, J. Pain 20 (6) (2019) 611–628.
15. G. Di Stefano, C. Celletti, R. Baron, et al., Central sensitization as the mechanism underlying pain in joint hypermobility syndrome/Ehlers-Danlos syndrome, hypermobility type, Eur. J. Pain 20 (2016) 1319–1325.
16. G.J. Macfarlane, M.S. Barnish, E. Pathan, et al., Co-occurrence and characteristics of patients with axial spondyloarthritis who meet criteria for fibromyalgia: results from a UK national register, Arthritis Rheumatol 69 (2017) 2144–2150.
17. O. Gendelman, H. Amital, Y. Bar-On, et al., Time to diagnosis of fibromyalgia and factors associated with delayed diagnosis in primary care, Best Pract. Res. Clin. Rheumatol. 32 (4) (2018) 489–499.

18 F. Wolfe, H.A. Smythe, M.B. Yunus, et al., The American College of Rheumatology 1990 criteria for the classification of fibromyalgia. Report of the Multicenter Criteria Committee, Arthritis Rheum. 33 (2) (1990) 160–172.

19 H. Cohen, Controversies and challenges in fibromyalgia: a review and a proposal, Ther. Adv. Musculoskelet Dis. 9 (5) (2017) 115–127.

20 F. Wolfe, D.J. Clauw, M.A. Fitzcharles, et al., The American College of Rheumatology preliminary diagnostic criteria for fibromyalgia and measurement of symptom severity, Arthritis Care Res (Hoboken). 62 (5) (2010) 600–610.

21 G.J. MacFarlane, C. Kronisch, L.E. Dean, et al., EULAR revised recommendations for the management of fibromyalgia, Ann. Rheum. Dis. 76 (2017) 318–328.

22 N. Arora, A. Gupta, S.B. Reddy, Antinuclear antibody and subserology testing in the evaluation of fibromyalgia: a teachable moment, JAMA Intern. Med. 177 (2017) 1369.

23 F. Atzeni, R. Talotta, I.F. Masala, C. Giacomelli, et al., One year in review 2019: fibromyalgia, Clin. Exp. Rheumatol. 37 (116) (2019) S3–S10.

24 S. Sieczkowska, G. Vilarino, L.C. de Souza, A. Adrade, Does physical exercise improve quality of life in patients with fibromyalgia? Ir. J. Med. Sci. 189 (1) (2019) 341–347.

25 J. Bidonde, A. Busch, C. Schachter, et al., Aerobic exercise training for adults with fibromyalgia, Cochrane Database Syst. Rev. 6 (2017) CD012700.

26 I.C. Alvarez-Gallardo, J. Bidonde, A. Busch, et al., Therapeutic validity of exercise interventions in the management of fibromyalgia, J. Sports Med. Phys. Fitness 59 (5) (2018) 828–838.

27 R. Gilliland, D. Hommer, Rehabilitation and fibromyalgia, Medscape (2019).

28 L.B. Taw, E. Henry, Acupuncture and trigger point injections for fibromyalgia: East-West medicine case report, Alternative Ther. 22 (1) (2016) 58–61.

CHAPTER 10

Upper Extremity Swelling

Dr. Subhadra Nori, MD

Case Presentation

A 69-year-old lady presented to the clinic with a history of right upper extremity (RUE) swelling of 3-month duration. She reports no pain but there is some discomfort because of the weight of the limb. And she reports being embarrassed because it is drawing attention from onlookers. The swelling started first on the upper arm and now includes the hand. Sometimes she feels slight warmth.

Past medical history: She has a history of breast cancer for which she had a partial mastectomy followed by radiation therapy 2 years ago. No history of diabetes or hypertension (HTN), Hx of hypothyroidism. No history of travel to foreign country.

Social history: She works as a home health aide and lives with family and two grown-up kids in a private house with no stairs.

Past surgical history: Tonsillectomy as a child. Aforementioned surgery 2 years ago.

Allergies: Penicillin

Medications: Vitamins, D, B12 antioxidants, and synthroid 75 mcg daily.

Vital signs: BP 130/70 mmHg, RR: 14/min, PR: 65 per min, Temp 97º F, Ht: 5'5", Wt: 140 lbs

Examination: WB, WN female in no AD and ambulates normally

Head, eyes, ear, nose and throat (HEENT)-extraocular movements (EOM) PERRLA, no ptosis, no pallor

General: Alert, oriented – 3, slightly anxious

Extremities: Entire length of RUE is swollen, no erythema slightly warm to touch, no tenderness. Edema was pitting in nature.

Measurements: 5 cm above antecubital fossa 29 cm
5 cm below antecubital fossa 18.5 cm

Motor examination: Power was 4/5+ in biceps, deltoid, triceps, brachioradialis forearm extensors and flexors and finger extensors and flexors.

Reflexes: 1+ and symmetrical in biceps, triceps, and brachioradialis

Sensory examination: Intact to LT in all dermatomes of the upper extremity (UE).

Laboratories: White blood cell (WBC) 7000 cells/mL, hemoglobin: 12.0 g/dL, complete blood count (CBC), SMA 18, and erythrocyte sedimentation rate (ESR)—normal.

X-ray of the left UE (LUE): No evidence of lytic or blastic lesions in humerus, radius ulnar, and wrist bones and digits.

Surgical report: Two years ago, patient was diagnosed with stage 2 intraductal breast carcinoma on R. A modified radical mastectomy and axillary lymph node dissection was done. She received radiation therapy and tamoxifen. No breast reconstruction was done.

General Discussion

This case is an example of lymphedema (LE) acquired secondary to breast cancer treatment. The approach to a patient with LE is unique. The initial focus should be to differentiate congenital from acute. The second focus should be to determine whether it is transient or persistent. The third focus should be to determine if any evidence of metastasis exists. The fourth is to determine the stage. Treatment of LE is held in two phases: (1) reduction of fluid and (2) maintenance.

Review of Proposed Pathology and Pathobiomechanics

LE is accumulation of protein-rich fluid (lymph) in tissues. It usually results from impaired lymphatic system. The lymph vessel function is impaired, thus by interrupting the drainage. Normally lymph vessels remove excess fluid from tissues and transport it back to circulation. Lymph capillaries are situated in the dermis, woven like a cobweb which then drains to the lymphatic vessels in subcutaneous tissues ultimately via the thoracic duct directly to the circulatory system (Fig. 10.1). Any disruption of this process can lead to LE. In addition, immune cells mature in the lymph system. Therefore the lymphatic system is one of the most important defense mechanisms.

Classification

LE can be classified as primary or secondary:

- Primary LE is caused by developmental abnormalities of the lymphatic system. Symptoms may develop at birth or later in life.
- Secondary LE is caused by an acquired condition causing damage to the lymph system. The most common causes are infection, injury, and removal of lymph nodes in the underarm, groin, pelvis, or neck for treatment of cancer and radiation. In developed countries, surgical removal of lymph nodes for cancer treatment is the most common cause.[1] Given that breast cancer is the most common cancer among women, breast cancer related LE (BCRL) is the most common type of LE.[1] Other cancers that can cause LE in lower extremities are uterine cancer, prostate cancer, lymphoma, melanoma, vulvar cancer, or ovarian cancer.
- The risk of LE increases with the number of lymph nodes affected. There is less risk with the removal of only the sentinel lymph node (the first lymph node in a group of lymph nodes to receive lymphatic drainage from the primary tumor).
- Lymphatic filariasis is caused by parasitic infection/infestation by microfilaria of *Wuchereria bancrofti* and affects over 120 million people in 72 countries, including parts of the Caribbean and South America. It is considered globally as a neglected tropical disease. Adult filarial worms commonly cause subclinical lymphatic dilatation and dysfunction. This condition is also known as elephantiasis. The chronic manifestations of LE and/or hydrocele will develop in approximately 30% of infected persons. LE mostly affects the legs, but can also occur in the arms, breasts, and genitalia. Most people develop these symptoms years after infection has cleared. Recurrent secondary bacterial infections of the affected extremity, characterized by severe pain, fever and chills, hasten the progression of LE to its advanced stage, known as *elephantiasis*[2,3] (Fig. 10.2).

Incidence of Lymphedema

BCRL is reported in 7% to 77% of patients who have undergone axillary lymph node dissection because of transection of lymph vessels.[4] Those with sentinel node biopsy had a much lower (3%–7%) incidence.[5,6] Other risk factors identified as causing BCRL are occupation, infection, increased BMI, age above 65 years, and radiation. Breast reconstruction was not considered a risk factor.[7,8]

Symptoms

The entire limb is swollen: upper limb on the same side of operation for breast cancer and lower limb in the other cancers mentioned earlier. Usually there is no pain unless infected. Patients may

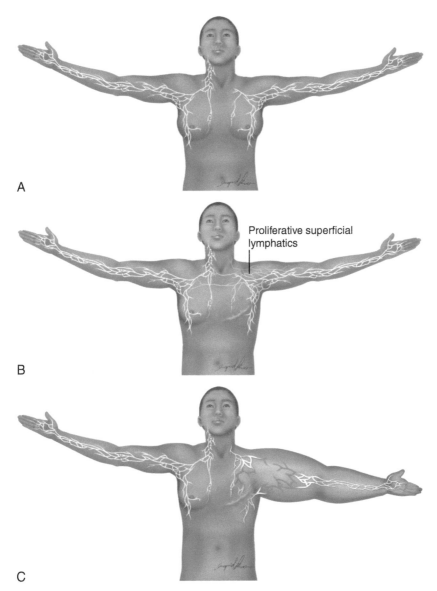

Fig. 10.1 (A) Normal lymph circulation. (B) Lymph node removal and mastectomy, with development of proliferative superficial lymphatics, hence no or minimal swelling. (C) Lymph node removal and mastectomy, without development of proliferative superficial lymphatics, hence significant swelling. (From M. Nitti, G.E. Hespe, D. Cuzzone, S. Ghanta, B.J. Mehrara, Principles and Practice of Lymphedema Surgery, Elsevier, Philadelphia, 2015, 40–50.).

also be depressed because of the appearance and unwanted attention drawn to them. They also complain of garments being tight.

Neurologic symptoms such as tingling, numbness, and muscle weakness because of entrapment of peripheral nerves in the UE or tumor involvement of the brachial plexus may be experienced. Radiation therapy usually affects the upper trunk and tumor affects the lower trunk of the brachial plexus.[9]

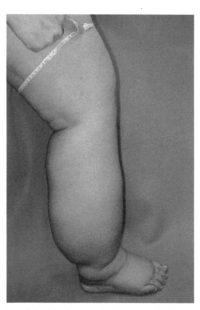

Fig. 10.2 Elephantiasis. (From M. Nitti, G.E. Hespe, D. Cuzzone, S. Ghanta, B.J. Mehrara, Principles and Practice of Lymphedema Surgery, Elsevier, Philadelphia, 2015, 40–50.).

Grading of Lymphedema (Table 10.1)

The following system is used to diagnose and describe LE based on size of the affected limb. Grades 1, 2, 3, and 4 are based on size of the affected limb and how severe the signs and symptoms are:

Stage I: The limb (arm or leg) is swollen and feels heavy. The edema is of pitting type.

Stage II: The limb is swollen and feels spongy. This is nonpitting and feels hard. There may be peau d'orange appearance (Fig. 10.3).

Stage III: This is the most advanced stage. The swollen limb may be very large. Stage III LE rarely occurs in breast cancer patients. Stage III is also called lymphostatic elephantiasis (see Fig. 10.2).

Another method is from the International Society of Lymphology.

Staging of Lymphedema Adapted From the International Society of Lymphology

Stage	Description	Characteristics
0	Latent	Some damage to lymphatics; no visible edema yet
1	Spontaneously reversible, acute phase	Pitting edema; reversible with elevation of the arm. Usually, upon waking in the morning, the limb(s) or affected area is normal or almost normal size
2	Spontaneously irreversible, chronic phase	Spongy consistency and is "nonpitting." Fibrosis found in Stage 2 lymphedema marks the beginning of the hardening of the limbs and increasing size

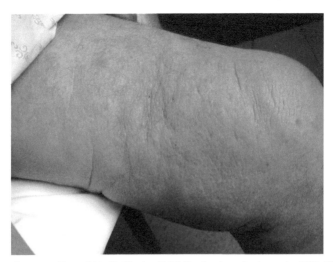

Fig. 10.3 Peau d'orange. (From A.K. Kurklinsky, T. W. Rooke, Lymphedema, in: W.S. Moore, Moore's Vascular and Endovascular Surgery, A Comprehensive Review, 9e, Elsevier, 2018, Fig. 56-1.)

Stage	*Description*	*Characteristics*
3	Elephantiasis; irreversible, end stage	Irreversible and usually the limb(s) is/are very large. The tissue is hard (fibrotic) and unresponsive; consider debulking surgery at this stage

Examination of the extremity includes:

- Inspection for any evidence of infection or ulceration
- Palpation to assess if it is pitting or nonpitting and to look for signs of infection, such as warmth, erythema. Corresponding areas should be palpated for lymph node enlargement.
- Circumferential measurements should be taken at the axilla, upper arm, forearm, wrist, and fingers and compared with the uninvolved side. Circumferential (>2 cm) and/or volume (>200 mL) differences between the affected and nonaffected extremity can be performed to confirm the diagnosis. These should be periodically recorded after treatment starts to log the progress.[1]
- Water displacement by immersing the limb in a large container filled with water gives an idea of volume and is considered gold standard.[10]
- Perometry is a computer-based study using an infrared optical electronic scanner to calculate the volume of the affected limb.[1]
- Reflexes should be obtained and compared with the other side. Sometimes if the limb is too swollen, reflexes may be difficult to obtain.
- Motor examination of all key muscles to rule in or out any peripheral nerve involvement.
- Sensory examination of the dermatomes subserving the involved limb again to r/o any peripheral nerve involvement.

Finally, look for evidence of Horner syndrome, which if present points to possible brachial plexus lower trunk involvement. This is because the sympathetic trunk is located in close proximity to the lower trunk. As mentioned, breast cancer metastases can spread to the lower trunk of the brachial plexus. Horner syndrome (or oculosympathetic paresis) results from an interruption of the sympathetic nerve supply to the eye and is characterized by the classic triad of miosis (i.e., constricted pupil), partial ptosis, and loss of hemifacial sweating (i.e., anhidrosis).

Causes of Horner syndrome include:

- Lesion of the primary neuron
- Brainstem stroke or tumor or syrinx of the preganglionic neuron—up to 33% of patients with brainstem lesions demonstrated Horner syndrome
- Trauma to the brachial plexus
- Tumors (e.g., Pancoast) or infection of the lung apex
- Lesion of the postganglionic neuron
- Dissecting carotid aneurysm—carotid artery ischemia
- Migraine
- Middle cranial fossa neoplasm[11]

Diagnosis

The diagnosis is usually established by history and clinical examination. Family history is important in assessing primary LE. History of trauma or surgery is essential. Care should be taken to include a comprehensive method of examining the patient as mentioned earlier.

Other diagnostic options are lymphoscintigraphy, ultrasonography, computed tomography, and magnetic resonance imaging.

Bioimpedence spectroscopy (BIS) is a new diagnostic tool to diagnose LE. It is a technique that assesses the extracellular fluid compartment before visible changes have settled. BIS mainly focuses on changes in electrical conductance of extracellular fluid.[12]

Lymphoscintigraphy is a nuclear medicine study of flow times. Technetium 99m sulfur colloid is injected intradermally, and the transit time to lymph node basins can be measured to see if it is slow or totally absent.[13]

Lymphography—radioopaque material is directly injected into peripheral lymph vessels. This technique is rarely done because of the risk of damaging lymph vessels.

Another option is magnetic resonance lymphangiography, a fairly new entity that involves the injection of gadolinium into the hand or foot to clarify the course of lymphatics. This aids in the detection of severity of LE while the anatomy of the lymphatic channels and the status of the soft tissues can also be depicted.[14]

Treatment

The mainstay of the treatment is reduction of edema and prevention of complications as infections. There is no absolute cure; however, effective treatment techniques are available.

These can be classified as nonsurgical and surgical.

COMPLETE DECONGESTIVE THERAPY

There are two phases of management: reductive (phase 1) and maintenance (phase 2). Complete decongestive therapy (CDT) is considered the gold standard treatment method in the management of LE.

REDUCTIVE PHASE

Volume is reduced by techniques, including manual lymph drainage and compression therapy using compressive devices such as pumps or manually. Physical exercise and proper skin care as self-management are essential components of this phase.

COMPRESSION DEVICES

Compression devices are pumps connected to a sleeve that wraps around the arm or leg and applies pressure on and off. The sleeve is inflated and deflated on a timed cycle. This pumping action may help move fluid through lymph vessels and veins and keep fluid from building up in the arm or leg. Compression devices may be helpful when added to compressive bandages or garments. Bandages are given for short-term and garments for long-term treatment therapy.

The use of these devices should be supervised by a trained professional because too much pressure can damage lymph vessels near the surface of the skin. Tubular bandaging then provides short stretch and "working pressure," which allows muscle contractions to direct interstitial flow.[15]

Maintenance Phase

After obtaining a reasonable volume reduction, elastic garments (elastic stockings/sleeves/gloves) and bandages are used. Elastic garments are socially more acceptable than bandages. These compression garments stretch in both length and width. Off-the-shelf garments do not fit everyone. Custom-made ones are tailored for individual use. These should be worn during the day. Many manufacturers are available. Some of the most widely used include Barton Carey, Godfried, Jobst, Juzo, Medi, and Sigvaris. They offer varied pressures from 18 to 60 mmHg. Patients with LE require the 60-mmHg range.

Care should be taken to rule out existence of conditions with acute inflammation, such as cellulitis, congestive heart failure, and acute-phase venous thrombosis because CDT is contraindicated in these situations.

This therapy must also be carefully selected in patients with sensory paralysis, neuroparalysis, or occlusive peripheral artery disease (contraindicated for limbs with severe ischemia).

Skin care—lymph is a protein-rich fluid and stagnation of lymph is a very good source of infections. Therefore it is of utmost importance to educate patients regarding hygiene and avoiding injury to skin. In some centers, a list of dos and don'ts is routinely provided.

MLD—in this procedure, soft stimuli are used to direct lymph flow from subcutaneous tissue of an affected limb and slowly induce it to the normally functioning lymphatic system. Treatment is focused on the subcutaneous tissue of an affected limb. Only soft compression should be used.

Exercises—both light exercise and aerobic exercise help the lymph vessels move lymph out of the affected limb and decrease swelling. Elevation of the limb especially at night should be encouraged. The aim of exercises is postulated that muscular movement inhibits leakage from capillaries, leading to edema improvement. Furthermore, the lymph vessel pressure improves the valve function, promoting lymph induction.[16]

Drugs—various drugs have been used.

Diuretics, in the initial phase, are effective in some patients by inducing diuresis. However, LE treatment is limited, and these agents may induce body fluid/electrolyte imbalance. Long-term administration is not shown to be helpful and should be avoided.

Benzopyrones—oral benzopyrones may hydrolyze tissue protein while activating the lymph transport route, promoting its absorption. Benefits are not seen. Hepatomegaly is a potential side effect.

Antimicrobial agents—antibiotics have a role in the management of LE if inflammation develops. After confirming hematologic findings of inflammation, such as leukocytosis and positive reactions to CRP, broad-spectrum antibiotics, including penicillin and cephems, should be administered, and CPT must be discontinued for resting. Antibiotic therapy should be discontinued if hematologic data normalize.

IMMUNOTHERAPY

Autologous lymph activated and infused into arteries may activate macrophages in the affected-limb interstitial tissue, decomposing an excess level of protein. However, its persistent effects remain to be clarified.

GENE THERAPY

Particularly in patients with primary LE, gene abnormalities were reported. Recent studies reported hepatocyte growth factor (HGF)–related neovascularization. Clinical studies of HGF were carried out to investigate peripheral vascular growth.[17]

LASER THERAPY

Low-level laser therapy (LLLT) has been shown to improve measurable physical parameters, as well as subjective pain scores.[18] It has been theorized that LLLT increases lymphatic drainage by stimulating the formation of new lymph vessels, by improving lymphatic flow, and by preventing formation of fibrotic tissue.[19]

Usually, LLLT is used in combination with CDT.

Surgical Options

Several reductive techniques and physiologic techniques are in use.

DIRECT EXCISION

In the technique called Charles procedure, there is complete removal of all subcutaneous tissue, lymphedematous tissue, and skin grafting.[20] This method, although it reduces volume, can be quite disfiguring. It requires blood transfusions and lengthy wound healing. Direct excision techniques may involve full-thickness skin grafting or vacuum-assisted closure therapy.[21] In extreme cases, these techniques can improve quality of life.

LIPOSUCTION

Liposuction involves surgical debulking and is shown to be effective for both congenital and acquired causes of LE. It is more effective in the UE. Liposuction has been shown to be very effective at reducing the volume to near normal.[22]

Lymphatic venous anastomosis, lymphaticolymphatic bypass, and lymph node transfer use recent developments in technology to assist in identifying lymphatic channels and lymph nodes.[23]

Summary

LE is a devastating disease because it is not easily cured. Treatment methods are uncomfortable and cause both physical and psychological morbidity to the patients. LE influences daily activities and affects patient self-esteem in various ways. Modern surgical and nonsurgical techniques offer numerous methods for the patients to overcome LE. Although many recent advances have been made, the treatment options require further research to be able to understand this devastating disease.

Key Points

- Lymphedema in this country is usually secondary to treatment of breast cancer.
- Lymphedema can lead to significant psychological and social impediments.
- Early diagnosis is important.
- Several management options exist, so careful selection is crucial for better outcomes.

References

1. Lymphedema: diagnosis and treatment, In: C.H. Thorne (Ed.), Grabb and Smith's Plastic Surgery, 7e, Wolters Kluwer Health, 2013, 980–988.
2. G. Dreyer, J. Noroes, J. Figueredo-Silva, New insights into the natural history and pathology of bancroftian filariasis: implications for clinical management and filariasis control programmes, Trans. R. Soc. Trop. Med. Hyg. 94 (6) (2000) 594–596.
3. J. Figueredo-Silva, G. Dreyer, Bancroftian filariasis in children and adolescents: clinical-pathological observations in 22 cases from an endemic area, Ann. Trop. Med. Parasitol. 99 (8) (2005) 759–769.
4. M. Noguchi, Axillary reverse mapping for breast cancer, Breast Cancer Res. Treat 119 (2010) 529–535.
5. W.P. Francis, P. Abghari, W. Du, C. Rymal, M. Suna, M.A. Kosir, Improving surgical outcomes: standardizing the reporting of incidence and severity of acute lymphedema after sentinel lymph node biopsy and axillary lymph node dissection, Am. J. Surg. 192 (2006) 636–639.
6. T. DiSipio, S. Rye, B. Newman, S. Hayes, Incidence of unilateral arm lymphoedema after breast cancer: a systematic review and meta-analysis, Lancet Oncol. 14 (2013) 500–515.
7. J.M. Armer, B.R. Stewart, Post-breast cancer lymphedema: incidence increases from 12 to 30 to 60 months, Lymphology 43 (2010) 118–127.
8. A.S. Gur, B. Unal, G. Ahrendt, et al., Risk factors for breast cancer-related upper extremity lymphedema: is immediate autologous breast reconstruction one of them? Cent. Eur. J. Med. 4 (2009) 65–70.
9. S.H. Kori, K.M. Foley, J.B. Posner, et al., Brachial plexus lesions in patients with cancer, 100 cases, Neurology 31 (1981) 45.
10. O. Kayıran, C. De La Cruz, K. Tane, A. Soran, Lymphedema: from diagnosis to treatment, Turk. J. Surg. 33 (2) (2017) 51–57.
11. C.M. Bardorf, Horner's syndrome, Medscape (2017).
12. B.H. Cornish, M. Chapman, C. Hirst, et al., Early diagnosis of lymphedema using multiple frequency bioimpedance, Lymphology 34 (2001) 2–11.
13. NLN Medical Advisory Committee, The Diagnosis and the Treatment of Lymphedema. Position Statement of the National Lymphedema Network, Feb, 2011. Available from: http://www.lymphnet.org.
14. L.M. Mitsumori, E.S. McDonald, P.C. Neligan, J.H. Maki, Peripheral magnetic resonance lymphangiography: techniques and applications, Tech. Vasc. Interv. Radiol. 19 (2016) 262–272.
15. H.N. Mayrovitz, The standard of care for lymphedema: current concepts and physiological considerations, Lymphat. Res. Biol. 7 (2009) 101–108.
16. A.L. Moseley, N.B. Piller, C.J. Carati, The effect of gentle arm exercise and deep breathing on secondary arm lymphedema, Lymphology 38 (2005) 136–145.
17. H. Shigematsu, K. Yasuda, T. Iwai, et al., Randomized, double-blind, placebo-controlled clinical trial of hepatocyte growth factor plasmid for critical limb ischemia, Gene Ther. 17 (2010) 1152–1161.
18. B. Smoot, L. Chiavola-Larson, J. Lee, H. Manibusan, D.D. Allen, Effect of low-level laser therapy on pain and swelling in women with breast cancer-related lymphedema: a systematic review and meta-analysis, J. Cancer. Surviv. 9 (2015) 287–304.
19. J. Robijns, S. Censabella, P. Bulens, A. Maes, J. Mebis, The use of low-level light therapy in supportive care for patients with breast cancer: review of the literature, Lasers Med. Sci. 32 (2017) 229–242.
20. R.H. Charles, Elephantiasis scroti, In: A. Latham, T.C. English (Eds.), A System of Treatment. III, Churchill Livingstone, London, 1912, 504–513.
21. G. Tahan, R. Johnson, L. Mager, A. Soran, The role of occupational upper extremity use in breast cancer related upper extremity lymphedema, J. Cancer Surviv. 4 (2010) 15–19.
22. H. Brorson, From lymph to fat: complete reduction of lymphedema, Phlebology 25 (Suppl. 1) (2010) 52–63.
23. D.W. Chang, Lymphaticovenular bypass for lymphedema management in breast cancer patients: a prospective study, Plast. Reconstr. Surg. 126 (2010) 752–758.

CHAPTER 11

Tingling and Numbness

Dr. Lynn D. Weiss, MD

Case Presentation

A 68-year-old male presents to the Physical Medicine and Rehabilitation (PM&R) clinic with a complaint of "pins and needles" in both feet. The sensation has gradually been getting worse over the past 2 years. He has no complaints of weakness. The patient describes the sensation as mildly painful (3/10) but it impedes his ability to walk comfortably.

Past medical history: History of diabetes for 20 years. He also has a history of obesity (BMI 31 kg/m^2), hypertension, and increased cholesterol. His medications include metformin, hydrochlorothiazide, and Lipitor.

Social history: He is currently retired. He used to work as a janitor for 41 years. He has smoked approximately one pack per day since the age of 16 years. He drinks about four to eight beers a day. He is independent in activities of daily living and ambulation. The patient lives with his wife in a ranch home with no steps. No other family members have had this type of problem.

Past surgical history: None.

Allergies: No known drug allergy.

Medications: Metformin 500 mg, two tablets twice a day, hydrochlorothiazide 25 mg twice a day, and Lipitor 20 mg once a day.

BP: 140/90 mmHg; RR: 15/min, PR: 72 per min, Temp: 98° F, Height: 5'8", Weight: 204 lbs, BMI: 31 kg/m^2.

PHYSICAL EXAMINATION

Well-developed male in no acute distress

Head, ear, eyes, nose, and throat (HEENT): Extraocular movements full, no ptosis.

General: He is alert and oriented. He is in no severe pain.

Extremities: No edema, no surgical scars.

MUSCULOSKELETAL EXAMINATION

Range of motion (ROM) of neck and back: Full range of motion in all directions.

MOTOR EXAMINATION

Bilateral upper and lower extremity strength 5/5.

There is no muscle wasting.

Deep tendon reflexes: 2+ in biceps, triceps and patella, 1+ in the ankle. Plantar response down going bilaterally. Negative Hoffmann.

SENSORY EXAMINATION

Decreased to light touch and pinprick in both legs distal to the ankle. Mild decrease to light touch and pinprick in the fingers distally and bilaterally. Proprioception impaired bilateral lower extremities. Decreased vibration sensation bilateral lower extremities.

Skin: No rashes or skin breakdown.

Pulses: Normal.

Gait: Within normal limits without any deviations. Tandem walks with mild difficulty.

Tone: Normal.

Cerebellar: Normal finger to nose.

Labs: Complete blood count (CBC) within normal limits, coagulation panel within normal limits, hemoglobin A1c (HbA1c) elevated at 8.9, complete metabolic panel elevated glucose 220, normal kidney parameters.

B12 and folate: Normal.

Serum protein electrophoresis (SPEP): Normal.
Heavy metal testing: Negative.
Chest x-ray: Negative for infiltrates or other lesions.
Electromyography (EMG): Distal sensory motor, axonal and demyelinating peripheral polyneuropathy, affecting the lower extremities more than the upper extremities. Distal lower extremity muscle abnormal spontaneous potentials (denervation) is noted. These findings are not in a myotomal or peripheral nerve distribution.

General Discussion

Patients with tingling and numbness in distal extremities bilaterally should prompt the clinician to consider peripheral polyneuropathy. Peripheral polyneuropathy can be either acquired or congenital. A pertinent family history asking about other family members must be included as part of the history. An assessment should be performed for peripheral polyneuropathy, as well as other causes for distal numbness. Note that peripheral polyneuropathy and other disorders can coexist. For example, patients with peripheral polyneuropathy are more prone to entrapment neuropathy, and peripheral polyneuropathy may exist in the setting of other disorders. In addition, it is important to assess the reason that patients has peripheral neuropathy, as that will affect the treatment plan.

When taking a history, ask patients about recent viral illnesses, any new medication they are taking, or if they have had any exposure to solvents or heavy metals.

Common Differential Diagnoses

1. **Diabetic peripheral neuropathy**—possible given the previous diagnosis diabetes, as well as poorly controlled blood sugars (as evidenced by elevated HbA1c levels).
2. **Alcoholic peripheral neuropathy**—patient has a long history of drinking alcohol. Alcoholic neuropathy can present after prolonged drinking.
3. **Toxic peripheral neuropathy because of chemicals**—patient worked as a janitor, and therefore might have been exposed to chemicals that are toxic to the peripheral nervous system (heavy metals, lead, mercury, arsenic, etc.).
4. **Peripheral neuropathy because of other causes**—could include undiagnosed thyroid disorder, human immunodeficiency virus (HIV), or other diseases.
5. **Malignancy**—Paraneoplastic syndrome can cause neuropathy. This is usually because of small cell carcinoma of the lung. This patient has a history of smoking, so is at increased risk for this type of neuropathy.
6. **Nerve entrapment proximally in the legs**—less likely given the symmetry of the symptoms, and the mild findings in the hands. Nerves can be entrapped anywhere in the legs. Common areas include:
   a. **Tarsal tunnel**—commonly cause numbness in the plantar surface of the feet and spare the dorsum of the feet.
   b. **Peroneal neuropathy at the fibular head**—commonly cause numbness on the top of the feet and spare the plantar surface of the feet.
   c. **Lumbosacral plexopathies**—less likely because these lesions are rarely bilateral and patients usually present with numbness in a peripheral nerve distribution (as opposed to a stocking/glove distribution). Motor function is also likely to be affected.
   d. **Radiculopathy**—less likely because the symptoms are bilateral and do not go above the ankles. Symptoms of radiculopathy would usually include back pain, motor weakness, and numbness in a nerve root distribution.
   e. **Spinal stenosis**—less likely because spinal stenosis usually presents with back pain (improved with flexion), as well as pain and numbness that does not go distal to the knees. Symptoms can be bilateral.

7. **Upper motor neuron lesion**—a central nervous system lesion is less likely given the distribution of the sensory impairment (distal and bilateral, affecting upper, as well as lower extremities), as well as normal tone, negative Hoffmann, and down-going plantar reflexes.

8. **Hereditary peripheral neuropathy**—less likely given the lack of family history but should not be excluded.

9. **Peripheral vascular disease**—is usually distal and may mimic the symptoms of peripheral polyneuropathy. However, pulses on this patient were normal.

10. **Diabetic amyotrophy**—can occur in diabetic patients. It frequently presents with the acute onset of unilateral pain and weakness (however, it may be bilateral). This is followed by severe atrophy. Affected nerves are usually more proximal than in a distal peripheral polyneuropathy. This patient did not have proximal pain, the onset was chronic, and there was no muscle wasting.

11. **Neuropathy as a side effect of medication**—numerous medications can cause peripheral polyneuropathy as a side effect, including some cancer medications, antialcohol drugs, anticonvulsants, immune suppression medications, antibiotics, and heart or blood pressure medications.

12. **Autoimmune inflammatory neuropathy**—includes Guillain-Barré syndrome (acute inflammatory demyelinating polyneuropathy [AIDP], as well as chronic inflammatory demyelinating polyneuropathy [CIDP]). Patients may report an antecedent viral infection. Usually, in Guillain-Barré, the symptoms are acute and ascending. Here, the symptoms were more chronic and limited to a distal distribution.

13. **Neuropathy caused by vitamin deficiency**—can be secondary to vitamin deficiency, especially vitamin B12 and folate. This may be seen in patients with alcoholism.

14. **Idiopathic neuropathy**—up to 46% of patients[1] develop peripheral polyneuropathy for which the reason is not clear.

15. **Small fiber neuropathy**—this type of neuropathy affects the small c fibers. Because nerve conduction testing only assesses for larger nerve fiber types, this type of neuropathy will yield a negative nerve conduction study (NCS)/electromyography (EMG).

Case Discussion

Our patient has several reasons to have a peripheral polyneuropathy, including diabetes, alcohol use, possible toxic chemical exposure, and smoking. He complains of numbness and tingling in the feet, but on physical examination, the hands are mildly affected as well. This is common in peripheral polyneuropathy because the nerves in the legs are longer and cooler than those in the arms. However, other diseases that can mimic peripheral neuropathy or coexist with peripheral neuropathy must be excluded.

The earlier EMG is helpful to further narrow down the differential diagnosis. Diabetic peripheral polyneuropathy typically presents as a distal sensory motor, axonal, and demyelinating peripheral polyneuropathy. The other main cause of this type of neuropathy is uremic peripheral polyneuropathy. Because kidney functions were normal, this is less likely. Distal denervation can be explained by the motor axonal component of the neuropathy. The patient's laboratory results further indicate that the most likely reason for the peripheral polyneuropathy is diabetes.

Review of Proposed Pathology

The exact mechanism of injury to the nerves in diabetic peripheral polyneuropathy is not clear. The toxic effects of hyperglycemia probably play a role.[2] Other factors include inflammatory, metabolic, and ischemic damage to the nerve.

CLINICAL SIGNS AND SYMPTOMS OF NEUROPATHY

Symptoms of peripheral polyneuropathy usually present in a "stocking and glove" distribution because of its distal prevalence. The feet are usually affected before the hands. Symptoms are rarely prominent proximal to the knees and elbows. Symptoms depend on the types of nerve fibers involved. Sensory symptoms may include numbness, tingling, pain, burning, and/or hyperesthesia or dysesthesia. If motor fibers are affected, distal weakness may be noted. The autonomic nervous system may also be affected, involving the cardiovascular system, gastrointestinal system, and sweat glands. Complaints might include abdominal pain, diarrhea, constipation, orthostatic hypotension, arrhythmias, syncope, voiding disorders, sweating disorders, and heat intolerance. Symptoms are usually gradual in onset. Patients may notice progressive difficulty walking or performing fine motor activities.

Physical examination findings will reflect the type and severity of nerve damage. Light touch and pinprick may be affected, as well as vibratory sensation. Balance may be decreased because of decreased proprioception. Deep tendon reflexes may be diminished, especially distally. If motor fibers are affected, strength may be decreased and muscle atrophy may be present (again, distal more than proximal). Autonomic dysfunction may be present as well. As patients may not be able to feel pain distally, it is important to look for skin breakdown, especially under the feet.

ELECTROMYOGRAPHY

EMG testing (especially the nerve conduction component of the test) can be used to differentiate peripheral polyneuropathy from other nerve involvement, including focal nerve entrapment syndromes (i.e., tarsal tunnel syndromes) and radiculopathy. It is also helpful in diagnosing nerve and muscle pathology that may coexist with the neuropathy. EMG can assess the type of neuropathy (axonal, demyelinating, or both; sensory, motor, or both; distal or proximal; uniform or segmental).

EMG testing can further help to prognosticate. The amount of conduction velocity slowing and increased distal latency indicates the severity of the demyelinating component. Dispersion of the compound motor action potential (CMAP) and sensory nerve action potential (SNAP) may also be noted, especially in acquired peripheral polyneuropathies. The reduction in amplitude indicates the severity of the axonal component. If distal denervation is severe, the motor units in that muscle are severely compromised. This indicates severe axonal damage and a poorer prognosis. Chronicity can be assessed by changes in the motor unit.

Other causes of peripheral neuropathy noted in the differential diagnosis can be excluded based on the findings of the EMG study (Table 11.1).[3] Alcoholic peripheral neuropathy usually presents as an axonal sensory motor neuropathy. Toxic neuropathies also usually present as axonal sensory motor neuropathies. Paraneoplastic syndrome peripheral neuropathy typically presents on EMG as a sensory axonal neuropathy. Entrapment neuropathies will typically demonstrate conduction velocity slowing across the area of entrapment or conduction block (neurapraxia). Radiculopathy will typically demonstrate normal nerve conduction studies, but may demonstrate denervation in a nerve root distribution. Spinal stenosis will typically show bilateral multilevel paraspinal denervation with few findings in the limb (but usually proximal findings more than distal findings). Upper motor neuron lesions will have normal nerve conduction studies and no denervation. There may be decreased recruitment in muscles affected by the central lesion. Hereditary neuropathies usually present with uniform demyelination as opposed to acquired neuropathies, where some segments have faster conduction velocities and some have slower conduction velocities.

IMAGING STUDIES

In this patient with a long history of smoking, it is reasonable to order a chest x-ray to rule out a malignancy. As noted earlier, small cell carcinoma can cause paraneoplastic syndrome, which presents as a peripheral neuropathy. Usually, paraneoplastic syndrome neuropathy is sensory axonal.

TABLE 11.1 ■ Polyneuropathy

"A PATIENT WITH TINGLING AND NUMBNESS"

EMG Finding	Polyneuropathy					
	Uniform Demyelinating Mixed Sensorimotor Polyneuropathy	Segmental Demyelinating Motor >Sensory Polyneuropathy	Axon Loss Motor >Sensory Polyneuropathy	Sensory Axon Loss Neuropathy	Axon Loss Mixed Sensorimotor Polyneuropathy	Mixed Axonal and Demyelinating Sensorimotor Polyneuropathy
CMAP amplitude	Normal	Decreased secondary to dispersion or conduction block	Decreased	Normal	Decreased	Decreased
Motor latency	Increased	Increased	Normal	Normal	Normal	Increased
Motor conduction velocity	Decreased	Decreased	Normal	Normal	Normal	Decreased
Dispersion of CMAP	No	Yes	No	No	No	No
SNAP amplitude	Normal	Normal or decreased	Decreased (usually)	Decreased	Decreased	Decreased
SNAP conduction velocity	Decreased	Decreased (somewhat)	Normal	Normal	Normal	Decreased
Needle EMG: Would fibs and PSWs likely be noted?	No (normal)	No (normal)	Yes	No (normal). Needle EMG assesses motor fibers only	Yes	Yes

Continued

TABLE 11.1 ■ Polyneuropathy—cont'd

| | Polyneuropathy | | | | | |
EMG Finding	Uniform Demyelinating Mixed Sensorimotor Polyneuropathy	Segmental Demyelinating Motor >Sensory Polyneuropathy	Axon Loss Motor >Sensory Polyneuropathy	Sensory Axon Loss Neuropathy	Axon Loss Mixed Sensorimotor Polyneuropathy	Mixed Axonal and Demyelinating Sensorimotor Polyneuropathy
Common diseases	1. Hereditary motor sensory neuropathy type I, III, VI (distal weakness with little atrophy) 2. Metachromatic leukodystrophy 3. Krabbe leukodystrophy 4. Adrenomyeloneuropathy 5. Congenital hypomyelinating neuropathy 6. Tangier disease 7. Cockayne syndrome 8. Cerebrotendinous xanthomatosis	1. AIDP: Guillain-Barré syndrome (ascending proximal weakness) 2. CIDP (weakness of asymmetric low extremities) 3. Osteosclerotic myeloma 4. Leprosy 5. Acute arsenic polyneuropathy 6. Pharmaceuticals (amiodarone perhexiline) high-dose Ara-C carcinoma, AIDS	1. Paraneoplastic motor neuronopathy (distal weakness) 2. Porphyria 3. Axonal Guillain-Barré syndrome 4. Hereditary motor sensory neuropathy types II and V 5. Lead neuropathy 6. Dapsone neuropathy	1. Paraneoplastic (sensory, painful in distal extremities) 2. Hereditary sensory neuropathy types I-IV 3. Friedreich ataxia 4. Spinocerebellar degeneration 5. Abetalipoproteinemia (Bassen-Kornzweig disease) 6. Primary biliary cirrhosis 7. Acute sensory neuronopathy 8. Cisplatin toxicity 9. Lymphomatous sensory neuronopathy 10. Chronic idiopathic ataxic neuropathy 11. Sjögren syndrome 12. Fisher variant Guillain-Barré syndrome 13. Paraproteinemias 14. Pyridoxine toxicity 15. Amyloidosis	1. Alcoholic polyneuropathy (distal symmetric weakness) 2. Vitamin (thiamine, B12) deficiency (distal symmetric weakness) 3. Gouty neuropathy 4. Metal neuropathy (e.g., mercury, thallium, gold) 5. Sarcoidosis 6. Connective tissue diseases (e.g., rheumatoid arthritis, SLE) 7. Gastrectomy, gastric restriction surgery for obesity 8. Chronic liver disease 9. Neuropathy of chronic illness 10. Hypothyroidism 11. Myotonic dystrophy 12. AIDS 13. Critical illness neuropathy 14. Lyme disease 15. Vincristine neuropathy 16. Toxic neuropathy (acrylamide, carbon disulfide, carbon monoxide)	1. Diabetic polyneuropathy (distal symmetric weakness) 2. Uremia (distal symmetric weakness)

AIDP, Acute inflammatory demyelinating polyneuropathy; AIDS, acquired immunodeficiency syndrome; CIDP, chronic inflammatory demyelinating polyneuropathy; CMAP, compound motor action potential; EMG, electromyography; fibs, fibrillation potentials; PSWs, positive sharp waves; SLE, systemic lupus erythematosus; SNAP, sensory nerve action potential.
(From J. Weiss, L. Weiss, J. Silver, Easy EMG a Guide to Performing Nerve Conduction Studies and Electromyography, 2e, Elsevier, Philadelphia, 2016.)

Here, the patient had a sensory motor, axonal, and demyelinating neuropathy. If the patient did have a pure sensory axonal neuropathy, it would be reasonable to order a chest computed tomography (CT).

Because there was no evidence of an axial component of pain, there is no need for magnetic resonance imaging (MRI).

LABORATORY TESTING

Patients should be assessed for disorders that can cause neuropathy, especially if the primary cause is not obvious. This may include HgA1c, blood urea nitrogen (BUN) and creatinine, B12, folate, SPEP, heavy metal assessment, thyroid assessment, HIV, and erythrocyte sedimentation rate (ESR).

DISCUSSION

In patients with distal numbness and tingling, peripheral polyneuropathy must be considered, but other disorders must be ruled out. In addition, it is extremely important to distinguish the type of neuropathy so that appropriate treatment can commence. There are a variety of causes of peripheral neuropathy. Whether the axon, myelin, or both are affected is important. It is also important to note if motor fibers, sensory fibers, or both are affected. Finally, it is important to note if the findings are distal more than proximal.

Once the type of neuropathy is diagnosed, treat the responsible underlying medical condition. In addition, symptomatic treatment can be initiated. This usually consists of pharmacologic therapy.

Prognosis depends upon the severity of the neuropathy. The more severe the neuropathy, the worse the prognosis. Usually axonal neuropathies have a poorer prognosis than demyelinating neuropathies.

Prevention of diabetic peripheral polyneuropathy is important. Diabetic neuropathy affects 10% of patients with diabetes at diagnosis. Some 40% to 50% of patients will develop diabetic neuropathy within 10 years of diagnosis.[4] Once the neuropathy is established, it is usually not reversible, even with strict glycemic control. Glycemic control has been shown to be more efficacious in type 1 than type 2 diabetics. Several studies have shown that enhanced glucose control can help to improve nerve conduction studies in both type 1 and type 2 diabetics and help prevent the development of clinical neuropathy in type 1 diabetics.[5]

If no cause can be determined for the peripheral polyneuropathy (especially in patients whose EMG is negative), skin biopsy and autonomic testing can be considered. Nerve biopsy can be indicated if vasculitis or amyloidosis is suspected.

TREATMENT

Pharmacotherapy

There are several treatment categories for peripheral neuropathy. These include:

Antidepressants—antidepressants (tricyclics and those that inhibit the reuptake of serotonin and noradrenaline) may alter the central perception of pain. These can include duloxetine, amitriptyline, and desipramine. The starting dose should be low and gradually increased until pain relief is achieved.

Anticonvulsants—these medications include pregabalin[6,7] and gabapentin. Pregabalin is thought to work by reducing substance P and glutamate levels and improving the release of norepinephrine. Gabapentin affects voltage-gated calcium channels. They are both considered membrane stabilizing agents. As with the antidepressant category of medications, the starting dose should be low and then gradually increased.

Topical creams—lidocaine patches have been prescribed with limited value.[8] Capsaicin cream is sometimes used to treat diabetic peripheral polyneuropathy. Although efficacious in treating the management of symptoms in postherpetic neuralgia, there is minimal evidence that it benefits patients with diabetic neuropathy.[9]

Opioids are rarely indicated for neuropathic pain.[10]

Foot Care

Care of the diabetic patient with peripheral polyneuropathy must include adequate foot care. Diabetic patients are at increased risk for complications (particularly ulcers) because of several mechanisms, including loss of sensory protection, vascular disease, and poor healing (secondary to vascular and metabolic factors). Patients should be seen periodically by a podiatrist and should be cautioned against cutting their own toenails. Proper foot care involves teaching patients how to inspect their foot, usually using a long-handled mirror to ensure viewing of the bottom of the foot. This can help prevent ulcers, skin breakdown, infection, and possible amputation. Specialized footwear with a high toe box may help prevent skin breakdown (especially if there is clawing or deformity of the toes). Patients should also be assessed for peripheral vascular disease.

Physical/Occupational Therapy

A trial of transcutaneous electrical stimulation (TENS) may help alleviate the symptoms of peripheral polyneuropathy.[11] In addition, in patients who have an unsteady gait because of the neuropathy, physical therapy with gait training and an assessment for assistive devices may be beneficial. If the peripheral polyneuropathy affects the upper extremities and the patient has difficulty with fine motor movements, occupational therapy and assistive devices may be helpful.

RECALCITRANT PAIN

If a patient fails to respond to the earlier measures, a combination of two different classes of medication can be tried. Patients who still fail to receive adequate pain relief can be considered for spinal cord stimulation.[12]

Summary

This patient presented with worsening symptoms of numbness and tingling in the feet. On physical examination, mild symptoms were also present in the hands. There were no findings of upper motor neuron disorder. The patient was referred for EMG. Testing confirmed the diagnosis of peripheral neuropathy, but also revealed the type of neuropathy (distal sensory motor, axonal, and demyelinating). Subsequently, he received pain management with pregabalin. The dose needed to be gradually increased until he was stable on a dose of 100 mg three times a day. He also was counseled on smoking cessation, diet, and alcohol use. He was given an exercise program to gradually increase endurance and cardiac response. At a follow-up visit 3 months later, the patient had diminished symptoms and improvement in his HbA1c.

Key Points

- Patients with tingling and numbness distally should be assessed for peripheral polyneuropathy. Electrodiagnostic testing can help differentiate the type of neuropathy, severity, and acuity, as well as identify coexisting neuromuscular disorders. The type of nerve fibers affected can help determine the underlying reason for the symptoms. Treatment should be targeted to reduce pain and address the specific underlying cause of the neuropathy.
- Treatment should be initiated to reduce symptoms. In patients with diabetic neuropathy, it is important to maintain euglycemia to control symptoms and prevent progression.

References

1. S.A. Gordon, J. Robinson Singleton, Idiopathic neuropathy, prediabetes and the metabolic syndrome, J. Neurol. Sci. 242 (2006) 9.
2. A. Schreiber, C. Nones, R. Reis, J. Chichorro, J.M. Cunha, Diabetic neuropathic pain: physiopathology and treatment, World J. Diabetes 6 (3) (2015) 432–444.
3. J. Weiss, L. Weiss, J. Silver, Easy EMG a Guide to Performing Nerve Conduction Studies and Electromyography, 2e, Elsevier, 2016.
4. B.C. Callaghan, A.A. Little, E.L. Feldman, R.A. Hughes, Enhanced glucose control for preventing and treating diabetic neuropathy, Cochrane Database Syst. Rev. (2012) CD007543.
5. C.L. Martin, J.W. Albers, R. Pop-Busui, DCCT/EDIC research group, Neuropathy and related findings in the diabetes control and complications trial/epidemiology of diabetes interventions and complications study, Diabetes Care 37 (2014) 31.
6. R. Freeman, E. Durso-Decruz, B. Emir, Efficacy, safety and tolerability of pregabalin treatment for painful diabetic neuropathy: findings from seven randomized control trials across a range of doses, Diabetes Care 31 (2008) 1448.
7. S. Derry, S. Straube, P.J. Wiffen, D. Aldington, R.A. Moore, Pregabalin for neuropathic pain in adults, Cochrane Database Syst. Rev. 1 (2019) CD07076.
8. V. Bril, J. England, G.M. Franklin, et al., Evidence-based guideline: treatment of painful diabetic neuropathy: report of the American Academy of Neurology, the American Association of Neuromuscular and Electrodiagnostic Medicine, and the American Academy of Physical Medicine and Rehabilitation, Neurology 76 (2011) 178.
9. S. Derry, A.S. Rice, P. Cole, T. Tan, R.A. Moore, Topical capsaicin (high concentration) for chronic neuropathic pain in adults, Cochrane Database Syst. Rev. 1 (2017) CD007393.
10. R. Chou, J.C. Ballantyne, G.J. Fanciullo, et al., Research gaps on use of opioids for chronic noncancer pain: findings from a review of the evidence for an American Pain Society and American Academy of Pain Medicine clinical practice guideline, J. Pain 10 (2009) 147.
11. R.M. Dubinsky, J. Miyasaki, Assessment: efficacy of transcutaneous electric nerve stimulation in the treatment of pain in neurologic disorders (an evidence-based review). Report of the Therapeutics and Technology Assessment subcommittee of the American Academy of Neurology, Neurology 74 (2010) 173.
12. C.C.M. de Vos, R.B. Zaalberg, et al., Spinal cord stimulation in patients with painful diabetic neuropathy: a multicenter randomized clinical trial, Pain 155 (2014) 2426.

CHAPTER 12

A Patient With Gait Difficulty

Dr. Maryam Hosseini, MD ▪ Dr. Michelle Stern, MD

Case Presentation

A 60-year-old male, who presents to the Physical Medicine and Rehabilitation (PM&R) clinic for difficulty with walking. He endorses two near fall episodes in the past 6 months, as well as difficulty when starting to walk and with turns.

Past medical/surgical history: Atrial fibrillation on anticoagulant (Afib on AC), diabetes, hypertension, lumbar stenosis s/p laminectomy, R Carpal tunnel release.

Allergies: Tylenol, Macrobid, contrast dye.

Medication: coumadin, metformin, Lopressor, Tamsulosin.

Family History: Noncontributory.

Social History: Patient lives at home with wife in a three-floor family house, with six steps to enter and 13 steps to third floor. The patient uses a rolling walker, as well as a cane for stairs and requires some assistance from his wife for the activity of daily living

Former smoker denies any alcohol (EtOH) or rec drug use.

PHYSICAL EXAMINATION

BP: 130/75 mmHg, sitting, standing 120/70 mmHg, RR: 14/min, PR: 70 per min, Temp; 97° F, Ht: 5'5" Wt: 130 lbs, BMI 21 kg/m².

Head, ear, eyes, nose, and throat (HEENT): Extraocular movement (EOM) full, no ptosis.

General: Alert, oriented and in no acute distress. Extremely fatigued.

Extremities: No edema, no skin rashes, no fasciculation seen.

MUSCULOSKELETAL EXAMINATION

Visual inspection: Muscular bulk appropriate for age with no focal weakness. No gross evidence of joint or tissue swelling.

Range of motion (ROM): Full passive range of motion in all major joints of bilateral upper extremities (BUEs). ROM of the neck: Complete in all directions.

NEUROLOGIC EXAMINATION

Mental status: AO×3, hypokinetic dysarthria, hypophonia, speech fluent, comprehension intact, masked faces.

Cranial nerves: EOM intact, pupils equal and reactive to light and accommodation, reduced facial expression, tongue midline.

Motor: 5/5 strength in b/l upper/lower extremities; cogwheeling bilaterally R>L in upper extremity.

Reflexes: 1+ in b/l upper and lower extremities.

Plantar reflex: Symmetrical, plantar downgoing.

Sensory: Intact to light touch to b/l upper/lower extremities.

Coordination: Negative Romberg, able to do finger to nose.

Pill rolling resting tremor, tone was normal.

Gait: A decrease in step length and height stooped posture and reduced arm swing. Short and shuffling gait with a tendency to fall backward, positive retropulsion test. Episodes of freezing and difficulty completing turns.

General Discussion

The initial focus in the general approach to a patient with gait dysfunction should be on history (falls in the past, activity limitation, time frame symptoms noted), past medical history, and physical examination. The physical examination should include a full neurologic exam, comprehensive musculoskeletal exam, and cardiovascular including peripheral arterial disease (claudication), and orthostatic hypotension. Medications should also be reviewed closely. It is important to differentiate between neurologic and musculoskeletal disorders, as well as from medical conditions affecting the neuromusculoskeletal system. Always keep in mind that gait disorders, especially in geriatric population, may have several causes.[1–3]

Watching the patient walk is important to examine the gait cycle. Monitor the number of steps in a period of time (cadence), comfortable walking speed, stride length (the distance between any two successive points of heel contact of the same foot) and stride width (the side-to-side distance between the line of a step of the two feet), and stride angle.[4]

Specific gait patterns associated with particular diseases can provide us with vital clues towards diagnosis (Table 12.1).

Common Differential Diagnoses

Antalgic gait/arthritic gait—a limp that develops in response to pain. This can be caused by osteoarthritis in the lower extremity, ankle sprains, foot stress fracture, and so on. Because of pain on weight bearing, to avoid pain; weight is quickly shifted from the affected leg to the other leg.[5,6]

Cerebellar ataxic gait—presents as an insecure wobbly, broad-based stance and gait. Stooped posture accompanied by a cautious walk with variable step length is noted. Midline lesions in

TABLE 12.1 ■ **Specific Gait Patterns and Their Association With Particular Diseases**

Type	Features
Antalgic/arthritic gait	To avoid pain, weight is put on the affected leg for as short a time as possible, resulting in a limp
Cerebellar ataxic gait	Broad based stance and gait, variable step length, insecure and wobbly
Sensory ataxia	Broad based, while walking in a dark or performing the Romberg test and eliminating the visual input, can lead to worsening imbalance
Cervical spondylotic myelopathy	Decreased speed walk, with shorter stride lengths and longer double support duration
Psychogenic gait disorders	Mimic a very insecure gait, temporary improvement or complete resolution of symptoms can be seen while the patient is distracted or thinks he or she is unobserved
Vestibulopathic gait	The legs are slightly spread, and stride length is slightly reduced, Unterberger test positive, deviation to the affected side
Apraxic/dysexecutive gait	Difficulty and hesitation in initiating the gait, short shuffling gait, and freezing
Choreatic gait disorder	Sudden involuntary movements in knee and hip flexors leads to dancelike swaying movements
Parkinsonian gait	Decrease in step length and height, stooped posture, and reduced arm swing, en bloc turn
Neuromuscular gait	Instability of the weight-bearing hip and causes the nonweight-bearing side to drop (Trendelenburg sign), excessive side to side trunk motion and a waddling gait
Spastic gait/unilateral	Extensor synergy pattern with knees extended, ankles plantar flexed and inverted, the ipsilateral arm is often flexed (circumduction)
Spastic gait/bilateral	Thighs adducted because of increased tone with scissoring across the midline

the cerebellar vermis can lead to truncal ataxia. Clinical findings include difficulty with finger to nose test, finding of positive Romberg test, and nystagmus.[7]

Proprioception loss—can lead to sensory ataxia. It can be seen in dorsal column lesions and sensory neuropathy. Without visual input, such as walking into a dark room, a significant worsening of imbalance can be seen. Therefore providing visual input or feedback mechanisms like foot slamming against the ground can be used as a compensatory strategy.

Cervical spondylotic myelopathy—the most common form of spinal cord dysfunction in people over 55 years of age. Usually patient presents with weakness in the lower extremities, accompanied by upper motor neuron signs (corticospinal and spinocerebellar tract dysfunction) and spasticity.[8–10]

Functional neurologic disorder/psychogenic gait disorder—can present with unusual and inconsistent neurologic findings along with insecure gait. The diagnosis of exclusion should be the approach to these patients. One important confirmatory finding is a total improvement of neurologic signs while being distracted.[11,12]

Unilateral/bilateral vestibular dysfunction—leads to vestibulopathic gait. Positive Unterberger's stepping test (asking the patient to step in place for 20–30 seconds) and because of lack of vestibular ocular reflex, one feels like walking in darkness with a propensity to fall.[13,14]

Higher-level gait disorder/apraxic gait disorder—basically a failure of motor programming because of frontal lobe dysfunction. Hesitation and difficulty in initiating the gait, short shuffling gait, and freezing are the characteristic features.[15,16]

Choreatic gait disorder—a manifestation of Huntington disease and tardive dyskinesia and levodopa-induced dyskinesia. Sudden involuntary movements in the knee and hip flexors lead to dancing like wormy movements.[17]

Parkinson gait—characterized by shuffling gait, decrease in step length and height. Reduced arm swing and stooped posture have been attributed to the imbalance. Significant difficulty while initiating steps, reaching obstacles and turns (en bloc turn) happens and can lead to falling. Multiple system atrophy (MSA) is a combination of parkinsonism and cerebellar signs with orthostatic hypotension.[18,19]

Neuromuscular gait disorder—happens in cases of myopathy and proximal muscle weakness. Weakness in pelvic stabilizer muscles leads to a drop of weight-bearing side (Trendelenburg sign) and side-to-side trunk motion (waddling gait). Knee hyperextension gait can be seen in quadriceps muscle weakness. Ankle dorsiflexors weakness leads to high steppage gait with excessive foot lifting off the floor during the swing phase.[5]

Unilateral/bilateral lesions—lesions in the corticospinal tract at any level can lead to spastic gaits. In cases of unilateral cerebral cortex lesion, circumduction is manifested as extended knees and flexed inverted ankle plantar flexors. In bilateral lesions, adducted thighs and scissoring gait can lead to spastic paraparesis.[20]

Case Discussion

Our patient states that he has been struggling with his walking, including difficulty initiating walking, difficulty with obstacles, and in turning with reports of near fall episodes in the past 6 months. Blood pressure medication or tamsulosin can cause orthostatic changes, which can lead to falls. Given he is on anticoagulation, he is at higher risk for subdural hematomas after a fall and fall prevention is crucial. His past history of diabetes mellitus (DM), atrial fibrillation (which increases risk of stroke), and spinal stenosis may lead to the consideration of a neuropathic or brain disorder, or a spinal cord disorder, but his examination suggests other causes. On his examination, he is noted to have full strength, normal deep tendon reflexes, and no distal sensory abnormalities. Neuropathy is less likely with normal sensory, motor,

TABLE 12.2 ■ Atypical Parkinsonian Syndrome Types

Atypical Parkinsonian Types	Features
Multiple system atrophy (parkinsonian type)	- Symmetric onset of bradykinesia, rigidity, tremor - Rapid progression - Autonomic dysfunction (orthostatic hypotension, bladder dysfunction, impotence)
Progressive supranuclear palsy	- Early falls within the first year or two - Stiff broad based gait with knees extended and arms abducted (drunken sailor) - Limitation of downgaze, progressive to upgaze and lateral gaze palsies
Corticobasal ganglionic degeneration	- Marked asymmetric involvement - Cortical symptoms: frontal syndrome, apraxia - Basal ganglia symptoms: tremor, rigidity, and dystonia
Lewy body disease (parkinsonian dementia)	- Dementia (fluctuating cognition and orientation) with parkinsonism - Recurrent visual hallucinations

TABLE 12.3 ■ Secondary Parkinsonism Causes

Secondary Parkinsonism	Features
Drug-induced parkinsonism	- Secondary to dopamine receptor blocking agents, such as the antipsychotic agents haloperidol, thiothixene, and risperidone
Vascular parkinsonism	- Symptoms predominate in the lower limbs (lower body parkinsonism) - Deep brain structure (basal ganglia, thalamus) involvement signs as spasticity, hemiparesis, and pseudobulbar palsy
CNS infectious sequelae	- Prion diseases, Creutzfeldt-Jakob disease, SSPE, HIV, postencephalitic
Wilson disease	- Copper deposition in basal ganglia - Kayser-Fleischer ring

CNS, Central nervous system; *HIV*, human immunodeficiency virus; *SSPE*, subacute sclerosing panencephalitis.

and deep tendon reflexes, and without upper motor signs, cord compression is unlikely. The patient examination notes include tremor, cog wheeling, and a shuffling gait, which is typical for parkinsonism.

The most common cause of parkinsonism symptoms is Parkinson disease (PD) and this can lead to progressive disability. It affects males 1.5 times more than females.[21] PD is a clinical diagnosis, without a specific imaging study or laboratory test to confirm the diagnosis at this time. Clinical features include pill-rolling, resting tremor, unilateral involvement which over time can develop to asymmetric bilateral symptoms, olfactory dysfunction, and beneficial positive response to levodopa support the diagnosis of PD.[22,23]

Atypical parkinsonian syndromes, especially early in the course, can be misdiagnosed as PD. These disorders include MSA, progressive supranuclear palsy (PSP), corticobasal degeneration (CBD), and dementia with Lewy bodies (DLB)[24,25] (Table 12.2).

Other most commonly confused entities with PD include secondary parkinsonism causes. These include drug-induced parkinsonism (DIP), vascular parkinsonism, central nervous system (CNS) infectious sequelae, trauma, toxin exposure (manganese, rotenone), and Wilson disease[26,27] (Table 12.3).

Objective Data

Complete blood count/complete metabolic panel are all within normal limits in our case, with an international normalized ratio (INR) in the therapeutic range. The diagnosis of PD is based upon its unique clinical features obtained from the history and physical examination. Essential criteria are defined as bradykinesia accompanied by rigidity and/or resting tremor.[28] Beneficial/unequivocal response to dopaminergic therapy medication is important to follow as a supportive criteria.[29,30] Brain imaging is not routinely used in PD diagnosis unless there is a high suspicion about other causes, including normal pressure hydrocephalus or cerebrovascular etiologies. Also when there are indicating signs toward atypical parkinsonism, imaging might be of use.[31,32]

Review of Proposed Pathology

PD is a complex neurodegenerative disease that causes both motor and nonmotor symptoms. The hallmark of PD is the degeneration of dopamine-producing neurons in the substantia nigra. Histopathologically, alpha-synuclein (αSyn) protein aggregation creates insoluble intracytoplasmic material called Lewy bodies (LBs), which are the hallmarks for neurodegenerative processes, and are found in dopaminergic neurons in substantia nigra.[33,34]

CLINICAL SIGNS AND SYMPTOMS OF PARKINSON

Parkinsonian gait known as *shuffling gait* presents as short steps, narrow-based with flexed knees and stooped posture. Four classic signs suggest a diagnosis of PD, including resting tremor, rigidity, bradykinesia, and postural instability. It is not necessary for all four to be present at the time of diagnosis.[30,35] Resting tremors should not be confused with essential tremor. Essential tremor occurs with movements, has a frequency of 8 to 12 Hertz (HZ), and can be alleviated by alcohol or propranolol. Parkinson's pill-rolling tremor has a frequency of 3 to 6 Hz and usually involves the forefinger and thumb.[36,37] Symptoms are oftentimes unilateral and when they progress to bilateral limbs, it has an asymmetrical pattern of involvement. PD is more likely to have a progressive prognosis with male gender, early-onset gait difficulty, and postural instability.

DISCUSSION

Gait disorders, especially in the geriatric population, may have several causes. Obtaining a complete history and performing a thorough physical examination, including gait analysis, will help for proper differential diagnosis. Based on the patient's symptoms and physical examination, PD is high on the differentials. PD has various presentations, including motor and nonmotor symptoms. Early diagnosis and medical management achieve better outcome, including maximizing functional ability. Dopaminergic medications are the most commonly used medication in the early stages of PD. Having a personalized rehabilitation program along with pharmacologic management will facilitate reaching maximizing the patient's functional goals.[38]

MEDICATION

Although no medication can cure PD, it can slow down the disease progress. A mainstay of treatment focuses on motor symptoms management through dopaminergic medication. Dopamine precursors (levodopa/carbidopa) are the most commonly used and recommended medication, but the long-term/dose-dependent side effects are associated with dyskinesias and the wearing-off phenomenon. Other drug therapy choices can be used depending on the stage of the disease and symptoms[39,40] (Table 12.4).

TABLE 12.4 ▪ Mechanism of Action of Commonly Recommended Medication for the Treatment of Motor Symptoms of Parkinson Disease

	Metabolism to Dopamine	Levodopa, Carbidopa
Dopaminergic agents	Dopamine receptor stimulator in moderate to advanced disease	Bromocriptine, Pamidronate, Pramipexole
	Blocks peripheral activity of catechol-O-methyltransferase (COMT) inhibitors	Entacapone
	Monoamine oxidase inhibitor (MAO-B inhibitor) and reduces dopamine metabolism in early disease	Selegiline, Rasagline
	Anticholinergic (blocks acetylcholine receptor) specially used for tremor	Trihexyphenidyl, diphenhydramine
Nondopaminergic agents	Antiglutamatergic (blocks acetylcholine receptor and NMDA)	Amantadine

NMDA, N-methyl-D-aspartate.

SURGERY

Neurosurgical intervention, including a neurostimulator placement in the subthalamic nucleus (STN) known as *deep brain stimulation* (DBS), might be considered in cases with resistant tremor and medically refractory to medication. Long-lasting benefit in overall motor symptoms has been reported.[40,41]

THERAPY

Rehabilitation is the cornerstone of the nonpharmacologic management of PD. The National Institute for Health and Clinical Excellence (NICE) published a guideline focusing on the importance of the availability of multidisciplinary rehabilitation, including physical therapy, occupational therapy, and speech therapy to improve the quality of life and maximize the functional ability in PD.[42,43] PD affects the basal ganglia/striatum, which has an exclusive role in motor learning (Fig. 12.1). Although studies suggest slower learning rates in comparison with the control group, they still demonstrate sufficient capacity to benefit from exercise.[44] Exercise has been proven to enhance the neurotransmitters' influences and potentially improves the functional ability.[45]

Gait and balance are largely affected, so treadmill training, balance training, and high-intensity resistance exercises accompanied by visual (laser lights), auditory (portable metronomic devices), and tactile feedback might be beneficial in gait initiation, freezing episodes, and respectively gait speed.[45–49] Rollator, walker, and cane can be helpful in balance issues.[50,51] On the other hand, consistent aerobic activity and stretching programs should be recommended. Flexibility program should focus on the following body areas: chest wall, shoulder and elbows, hamstrings, calves, front of wrists and palms, low back and neck with strengthening of abdominals, quads, gluteals, back, and triceps. Different equipment, including shower chairs, raised toilet seats, with armrests and grab bars may be used as assistive devices.

The "Think Big" training features repetition and self-cueing for large-amplitude movements, such as arm swing or step. Walking tips for patients are to try to land with the heel first, thinking of each step as a big kick, focus on the size of the steps rather the speed of your steps, and avoid carrying many things while walking.[52,53]

In summary, PD can present with a gait disorder, especially in the older population. It is associated with motor and nonmotor symptoms that need to be evaluated and treated. Tremor, bradykinesia, postural instability, and rigidity are important to look for on examination.[46]

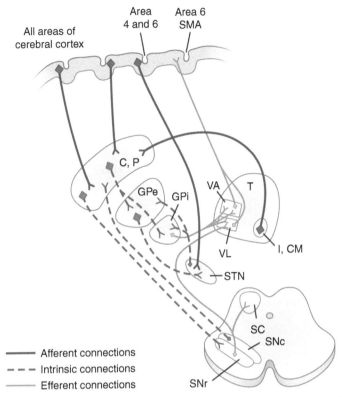

Fig. 12.1 Schematic drawing of interconnections between the basal ganglia and its afferent and efferent connections. *CM,* Centromedian nucleus of thalamus; *C,P,* caudate, putamen (striatum); *GPe,* lateral (external) globus pallidus; *GPi,* medial (internal) globus pallidus; *SC,* superior colliculus; *STN,* subthalamic nucleus; *SNc,* substantia nigra pars compacta; *SNr,* substantia nigra pars reticulata; *T,* thalamus; *VA,* ventral anterior; *VL,* ventrolateral. (From R.B. Daroff, J. Jankovich, J. Mazziotta, S. Pommeroy, Bradley's Neurology in Clinical Practice, 7e, Elsevier, Philadelphia, 2016, 1422–1466, Fig. 96.1.)

Key Points

- Gait disorder has many causes, both neurologic and nonneurologic. Careful attention to examination is needed to determine the etiology of a gait disorder. Follow-up on a diagnosis for Parkinson should be ongoing because there is no test specific for the diagnosis and can be misdiagnosed by other syndromes.

References

1. N.B. Alexander, A. Goldberg, Gait disorders: search for multiple causes, Cleve. Clin. J. Med. 72 (7) (2005) 589–590 596.
2. A.H. Snijders, B.P. van de Warrenburg, N. Giladi, B.R. Bloem, Neurological gait disorders in elderly people: clinical approach and classification, Lancet Neurol. 6 (1) (2007) 63–74.
3. N.C. Voermans, A.H. Snijders, Y. Schoon, B.R. Bloem, Why old people fall (and how to stop them), Pract. Neurol. 7 (3) (2007) 159–171.
4. R.W. Bohannon, A. Williams Andrews, Normal walking speed: a descriptive meta-analysis, Physiotherapy 97 (3) (2011) 182–189.
5. M.R. Lim, A. Wu, F.P. Girardi, F.P. Cammisa, Elderly patient with an abnormal gait, J. Am. Acad. Orthop. Surg. 129 (3) (2007) 81–95.

6. P. Mahlknecht, S. Kiechl, B.R. Bloem, et al., Prevalence and burden of gait disorders in elderly men and women aged 60-97 years: a population-based study, PloS One 8 (7) (2013) e69627.

7. S.M. Morton, A.J. Bastian, Relative contributions of balance and voluntary leg-coordination deficits to cerebellar gait ataxia, J. Neurophysiol. 89 (4) (2003) 1844–1856.

8. J.P. Kuhtz-Buschbeck, K. Jöhnk, S. Mäder, H. Stolze, M. Mehdorn, Analysis of gait in cervical myelopathy, Gait Posture 9 (3) (1999) 321–326.

9. A. Malone, D. Meldrum, C. Bolger, Gait impairment in cervical spondylotic myelopathy: Comparison with age- and gender-matched healthy controls, Eur. Spine J. 21 (12) (2012) 2456–2466.

10. H. Nishimura, K. Endo, H. Suzuki, H. Tanaka, T. Shishido, K. Yamamoto, Gait analysis in cervical spondylotic myelopathy, Asian Spine J 9 (3) (2015) 321–326.

11. L. Sudarsky, Psychogenic gait disorders, Semin. Neurol. 26 (3) (2006) 351–356.

12. T. Lempert, T. Brandt, M. Dieterich, D. Huppert, How to identify psychogenic disorders of stance and gait - A video study in 37 patients, J. Neurol. 238 (3) (1991) 140–146.

13. T. Brandt, M. Strupp, J. Benson, M. Dieterich, Vestibulopathic gait. Walking and running, Adv. Neurol. 87 (2001) 167–172.

14. H. Ling, Clinical approach to progressive supra-nuclear palsy, J Mov. Disord. 9 (1) (2016) 3–13.

15. P.D. Thompson, J.G. Nutt, Higher level gait disorders, J. Neural. Transm. 114 (10) (2007) 1305–1307.

16. J.G. Nutt, Higher-level gait disorders: an open frontier, Mov. Disord. 28 (11) (2013) 1560–1565.

17. Y.M.A. Grimbergen, M.J. Knol, B.R. Bloem, B.P.H. Kremer, R.A.C. Roos, M. Munneke, Falls and gait disturbances in Huntington's disease, Mov. Disord. 159 (2008) 251–260.

18. B. Bloem, Y. Grimbergen, J. Vandijk, M. Munneke, The "posture second" strategy: a review of wrong priorities in Parkinson's disease, J. Neurol. Sci. 248 (1–2) (2006) 196–204.

19. B.R. Bloem, J.M. Hausdorff, J.E. Visser, N. Giladi, Falls and freezing of gait in Parkinson's disease: a review of two interconnected, episodic phenomena, Mov. Disord. 19 (8) (2004) 871–884.

20. W. Pirker, R. Katzenschlager, Gait disorders in adults and the elderly: a clinical guide, Wien Klin. Wochenschr. 129 (3) (2017) 81–95.

21. L.M.L. De Lau, P.C.L.M. Giesbergen, M.C. De Rijk, A. Hofman, P.J. Koudstaal, M.M.B. Breteler, Incidence of parkinsonism and Parkinson disease in a general population: The Rotterdam Study, Neurology 63 (7) (2004).

22. C.D. Marsden, The mysterious motor function of the basal ganglia: the Robert Wartenberg Lecture, Neurology 32 (5) (1982) 514–539.

23. M.C. Rodriguez-Oroz, M. Jahanshahi, P. Krack, et al., Initial clinical manifestations of Parkinson's disease: features and pathophysiological mechanisms, Lancet Neurol. 8 (12) (2009) 1128–1139.

24. N.R. Mcfarland, Diagnostic approach to atypical parkinsonian syndromes, Contin. Lifelong Learn Neurol. 22 (4) (2016) 1117–1142.

25. A.B. Deutschländer, O.A. Ross, D.W. Dickson, Z.K. Wszolek, Atypical parkinsonian syndromes: a general neurologist's perspective, Eur. J. Neurol. 25 (1) (2018) 41–58.

26. M.V.G. Alvarez, V.G.H. Evidente, Understanding drug-induced parkinsonism: Separating pearls from oysters, Neurology 70 (8) (2008) e32–34.

27. J. Winikates, J. Jankovic, Clinical correlates of vascular parkinsonism, Arch. Neurol. 56 (1) (1999) 96–102.

28. D. Berg, R.B. Postuma, C.H. Adler, et al., MDS research criteria for prodromal Parkinson's disease, Mov. Disord. 30 (12) (2015) 1600–1611.

29. A.J. Hughes, S.E. Daniel, L. Kilford, A.J. Lees, Accuracy of clinical diagnosis of idiopathic Parkinson's disease: A clinico-pathological study of 100 cases, J. Neurol. Neurosurg. Psychiatry 55 (3) (1992) 181–184.

30. O. Suchowersky, S. Reich, J. Perlmutter, T. Zesiewicz, G. Gronseth, W.J. Weiner, Appendix A: Practice parameter: diagnosis and prognosis of new onset Parkinson disease (an evidence-based review): Report of the Quality Standards Subcommittee of the American Academy Neurology, Contin. Lifelong Learn Neurol. 67 (12) (2007) 2266.

31. A.J. Stoessl, W.R.W. Martin, M.J. McKeown, V. Sossi, Advances in imaging in Parkinson's disease, Lancet Neurol. 10 (11) (2011) 987–1001.

32. M. Politis, Neuroimaging in Parkinson disease: from research setting to clinical practice, Nat. Rev. Neurol. 10 (12) (2014) 708–722.

33. D.W. Dickson, Parkinson's disease and parkinsonism: neuropathology, Cold Spring Harb. Perspect. Med. 2 (8) (2012) a009258.
34. D.W. Dickson, H. Fujishiro, C. Orr, et al., Neuropathology of non-motor features of Parkinson disease, Park. Relat. Disord. 15 (3) (2009) S1–S5.
35. J. Massano, K.P. Bhatia, Clinical approach to Parkinson's disease: features, diagnosis, and principles of management, Cold Spring Harb. Perspect. Med. 2 (6) (2012) a008870.
36. H.J. Lee, W.W. Lee, S.K. Kim, et al., Tremor frequency characteristics in Parkinson's disease under resting-state and stress-state conditions, J. Neurol. Sci. 362 (2016) 272–277.
37. M.A. Thenganatt, E.D. Louis, Distinguishing essential tremor from Parkinson's disease: bedside tests and laboratory evaluations, Expert Rev. Neurother. 12 (6) (2012) 667–696.
38. M.E. McNeely, G.M. Earhart, Medication and subthalamic nucleus deep brain stimulation similarly improve balance and complex gait in Parkinson disease, Park. Relat. Disord. 19 (1) (2013) 86–91.
39. B.S. Connolly, A.E. Lang, Pharmacological treatment of Parkinson disease: a review, J. Am. Med. Assoc. 311 (16) (2014) 1670–1683.
40. P. Rizek, N. Kumar, M.S. Jog, An update on the diagnosis and treatment of Parkinson disease, CMAJ 188 (16) (2016) 1157–1165.
41. J. Voges, A. Koulousakis, V. Sturm, Deep brain stimulation for Parkinson's disease, Acta. Neurochir. Suppl. 2 (6) (2007) 20–28.
42. National Collaborating Centre for Chronic Conditions, Parkinson's disease. Diagnosis and management in primary and secondary care, Natl. Inst. Heal. Clin. Excell. Clin. Guidel. 35 (2006).
43. National Collaborating Centre for Chronic Conditions, Parkinson's Disease: National Clinical Guideline for Diagnosis and Management in Primary and Secondary Care, Natl. Inst. Heal. Clin. Excell. Clin. Guidel. (2006).
44. G. Abbruzzese, R. Marchese, L. Avanzino, E. Pelosin, Rehabilitation for Parkinson's disease: current outlook and future challenges, Park. Relat. Disord. 22 (1) (2016) S60–S64.
45. C.J. Hass, T.A. Buckley, C. Pitsikoulis, E.J. Barthelemy, Progressive resistance training improves gait initiation in individuals with Parkinson's disease, Gait Posture 35 (4) (2012) 660–674.
46. P.H. Chen, R.L. Wang, D.J. Liou, J.S. Shaw, Gait disorders in Parkinson's disease: assessment and management, Int. J. Gerontol. 7 (4) (2013) 189–194.
47. J. Mehrholz, J. Kugler, A. Storch, M. Pohl, K. Hirsch, B. Elsner, Treadmill training for patients with Parkinson's disease, Cochrane Database Syst. Rev. 22 (8) (2015) CD007830.
48. S.J. Lee, J.Y. Yoo, J.S. Ryu, H.K. Park, S.J. Chung, The effects of visual and auditory cues on freezing of gait in patients with Parkinson disease, Am. J. Phys. Med. Rehabil. 91 (1) (2012) 2–11.
49. S. Donovan, C. Lim, N. Diaz, et al., Laserlight cues for gait freezing in Parkinson's disease: an open-label study, Park. Relat. Disord. 17 (4) (2011) 240–245.
50. E. Cubo, C.G. Moore, S. Leurgans, C.G. Goetz, Wheeled and standard walkers in Parkinson's disease patients with gait freezing, Park. Relat. Disord. 10 (1) (2003) 9–14.
51. R. Boonsinsukh, V. Saengsirisuwan, P. Carlson-Kuhta, F.B. Horak, A cane improves postural recovery from an unpracticed slip during walking in people with Parkinson disease, Phys. Ther. 92 (9) (2012) 1117–1129.
52. L. Rochester, D. Rafferty, C. Dotchin, O. Msuya, V. Minde, R.W. Walker, The effect of cueing therapy on single and dual-task gait in a drug naïve population of people with Parkinson's disease in Northern Tanzania, Mov. Disord. 25 (7) (2010) 206–209.
53. S.V. Sarma, M.L. Cheng, U. Eden, Z. Williams, E.N. Brown, E. Eskandar, The effects of cues on neurons in the basal ganglia in Parkinson's disease, Front. Integr. Neurosci. 6 (2012) 40.
54. M.E. Tinetti, D.I. Baker, G. McAvay, et al., A multifactorial intervention to reduce the risk of falling among elderly people living in the community, N. Engl. J. Med. 331 (1994) 821.
55. M.C. Nevitt, S.R. Cummings, Type of fall and risk of hip and wrist fractures: the study of osteoporotic fractures, The Study of Osteoporotic Fractures Research Group, J. Am. Geriatr. Soc. 41 (1993) 1226.

INDEX

Page numbers followed by the letters b, f, or t indicate boxes, figures, and tables, respectively.